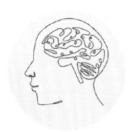

THE ADULT

Speech Therapy Workbook

WRITTEN & ILLUSTRATED BY
CHUNG HWA BREWER, MA, CCC-SLP

EDITED BY MIWA APARO, MOT

Published by Harmony Road Design LLC.

Copyright © 2021 Chung Hwa Brewer. All rights reserved.

No portion of this book may be reproduced in any form without permission from the author, except as permitted by U.S. copyright law. For permissions, email: contact@theadultspeechtherapyworkbook.com.

DISCLAIMER:

The advice and strategies found within this book may not be suitable for every situation. This work is sold with the understanding that neither the author nor the publisher are held responsible for the results accrued from the advice in this book.

This book is not intended to be a substitute for professional medical advice. The reader should always seek the advice of their physician, speech-language pathologist, and/or other qualified health care provider in any matters relating to their health.

FINANCIAL DISCLOSURE:

At the time of publication, the author and editor have a financial relationship with etsy.com/shop/harmonyroaddesign, theadultspeechtherapyworkbook.com, The Home Health SLP Handbook, and MedBridge. All other cited or recommended resources have no financial or non-financial relationship with the author or the editor.

ACKNOWLEDGEMENTS:

Thank you to my friends at UH for your support. A big thank you to my home health colleagues for replying to all of my texts and for sharing your knowledge. To my patients and their families, you do incredible work; thank you for your trust in me and for teaching me how to be a better person. Thanks, mom and dad, for being my workbook guinea pigs. And to Miwa, thank you for all the things.

ISBN

978-1-7338633-3-9

Also by the author:

The Home Health SLP Handbook (2019)

TheAdultSpeechTherapyWorkbook.com (co-author)

A to Z: A Speech-Language Pathology Alphabet (2018)

Cover art and design and page layout are by the author.

INTRODUCTION

Hello reader! This workbook was designed to be the go-to resource for speech therapists new to adult speech therapy. Equipped with these hundreds of pages of effective and practical treatment activities, I hope that you'll feel confident and prepared every time you greet a patient.

Visit **theadultspeechtherapyworkbook.com** for The Digital Adult Speech Therapy Workbook, Assessment Templates, Goal Banks, and Documentation Guides. You'll also find free patient worksheets, color photos for aphasia treatment, in-depth instructions for specific treatment approaches, and much more.

HOW THIS BOOK IS ORGANIZED.
- Each chapter begins with therapist instructions. These include how to use handouts and other treatment tips.
- Pages that are "For Therapist Eyes Only" have a gray background or header.
    - All of the other pages in this workbook are for direct patient or caregiver use.
- For the purposes of this book:
    - "Handouts" are informational pages, like swallowing strategies and tips on increasing comprehension.
    - "Worksheets" are the tasks that your patients complete, like balancing a checkbook and writing sentences.

ABOUT THIS WORKBOOK.
- Adult speech therapy: Techniques and tips for the most common diagnoses and disorders across all adult speech therapy settings.
- Evidence-based: Only the best for our patients. Please peruse the 100+ references at the end of the book!
- Practical: Functional, real-life tasks that work for patients.
- Copy and go: Easy-to-copy pages.
- Large and clear fonts: Easy to read for patients with lower vision and cognitive deficits.
- Treatment from Day 1: Tasks and handouts you can use on the very first day of therapy.
- Continued therapy: The handouts and tasks range from simple to complex activities and can be used as part of a home program.

COPYING & PRINTING.
- Copy pages directly or have a printshop (OfficeMax, etc.) spiral-bind the pages.

SUGGESTIONS.
- Focus on 2-3 handouts at a time with each patient.
- Review each handout with your patient.
- Highlight the information specifically important to your patient.
- Refer back to the handouts often.
- Mix the pen-and-paper worksheets with other functional tasks (also included in this book).

PATIENT-CENTERED TREATMENT.
- The World Health Organization defines health as more than the "absence of disease" *(ASHA, 2021c)*.
- Always consider your patient's quality of life when designing their treatment. What matters to them? In their environments? Their personal lives? Their relationships?

This workbook will complement your knowledge and skills, but it's not a comprehensive guide to speech therapy. It's assumed that you're a licensed therapist who earned a degree from an accredited speech therapy program.

Remember that a worksheet will only take a patient so far: It's your training and unique talents that will help your patients achieve a higher quality of life.

Questions? Visit theadultspeechtherapyworkbook.com or e-mail me directly at chung@theadultspeechtherapyworkbook.com.

Wishing you ther-happy days!
-Chung Hwa

CONTENTS

Refer to the beginning of each chapter for additional page numbers

WRITING GOALS 8

HOMEWORK LOG 12

DYSPHAGIA 13
- Neuroplasticity 24
- Safe Swallowing 33
- Effortful Swallow 34
- Puréed Diet 48
- Esophageal Diet 52
- Thickened Liquids 54
- Deep Breathing 57
- Head and Neck Stretches 61
- Tracheostomy Care 64
- Speaking Valve 67

MEMORY 81

Mild Memory Deficits
- Memory Strategies 92
- Ways to Improve Memory 93
- Memorize Lists 146
- Brain Organization Tips 155
- Remembering Instructions 156
- Remembering Reading Material 165

Moderate Memory Deficits
- How to Avoid Memory Loss 91
- Remembering Your Medications 114
- Monthly Calendar 120
- Remembering People's Names 134
- Remembering Appointments 158
- Memos & Appointments 161

Severe Memory Deficits
- Orientation 98
- Spaced Retrieval 99
- Memory Books 101
- Daily Journal 117
- Daily Schedule 119

PROBLEM SOLVING 177
Restorative Treatment
- Task Analysis 183
- TEACH-M 184
- Setting Goals 193
- Practical Math 202
- Sequencing 211
- Everyday Math 228

Compensatory Treatment
- Filling a Pill Box 192
- Organize your Bills 196
- Medical Alert Systems 197
- Medical Team Phone Numbers 209
- Meal Planning 218

VISUAL NEGLECT 247
Visual Scanning
- Lighthouse Technique 255
- Reading Strategies 256
- Reading Maps 285

Feedback Training
- Environmental Modifications 254
- Cancellation Task 258

APHASIA 295
- Cueing Hierarchy 301
- Communication Tips 313
- Language Expression & Writing 316
- Language Comprehension & Reading .. 361

MOTOR SPEECH 433
Restorative Treatment
- Sound Production Treatment 440
- Diaphragmatic Breathing 448
- Breath Control 450
- Sentence Stress 458
- Heteronyms 461
- Phonemic Lists 464

Compensatory Treatment
- Clear Speech Strategies 446
- Phone Calls 454

Conversation	455
Interview	456
Monologues	457

VOICE & RESONANCE ... 529

Resonance Treatment
Hypernasality	537
Nasal Air Emission	538
Cul-de-Sac Resonance	539

Voice Treatment
Vocal Tension	540
Vocal Weakness	541
Vocal Hygiene	551
Circumlaryngeal Massage	552

AAC ... 555
Listener Tips	564
Alphabet Board	569

FLUENCY ... 573
Fluency Strategies	579
Breath Curve	581

REFERENCES ... 583

ABOUT THE AUTHOR ... 589

Writing Goals

WHAT IS AN EXCELLENT GOAL.
- It's **appropriate** and **relevant** for your patient, given their unique situation
- It's the **right level of challenge**—not too hard and not too easy
- It's **specific**
- It's **measurable**
- It's achievable within an **appropriate time frame**
- It's insurance friendly (useful for most!)

SPECIFIC. Your goal should focus on an issue that the evaluation determined is a significant area of concern for the patient.
- Specific
    - "Safely swallow teaspoon amounts of thin liquids"
    - "Write at the sentence level"
    - "Complete simple short-term memory tasks"
    - "Produce multisyllabic words containing /k/ final"
- Not Specific
    - "Drink liquids." How much? What type of liquids?

ACCURACY LEVEL. Typically 70-90% accuracy.
- Less than 70% can be ineffective in helping patients reach goals while above 90% accuracy denotes mastery which often isn't our role (errorless learning and safety goals, including swallowing safety, are exceptions).

AMOUNT OF CUES. Measured by percentages, time units, and/or frequency per question or set of questions. Test your patient's stimulability to cues. This will help you decide the best cues to use for their specific goals.
- Cues per set of questions
    - **Minimal** is 1-25% of the time
    - **Moderate** is 26-50% of the time
    - **Maximal** is 51-75% of the time
    - **Dependent** is 76% or more of the time

Page 1 of 4

- Cues per each question may be a more subjective way of measuring cues. The amount of cueing you record depends on your professional judgment.
    - **Minimal** (first cue): You help the patient take the first step toward completing the task.
        - *For example, your patient is attempting to calculate the cost of an item after tax. Your minimal cue is, "What does 8% translate to in decimals?"*
    - **Moderate** (second cue): You help the patient take the next step toward completing the task. Either by answering your minimal cue question or by giving more information. You may need to give several moderate cues for each question, depending on how complex the task is.
        - *"The decimal amount is 0.08 and the item costs $75. How much money is 8% of 75?"*
    - **Maximal** (final cue): You help the patient take the final step toward completing the task. Either by answering your moderate cue question or giving more information.
        - *"The tax is $6. What is the total price of the item after tax?"*
- Cues per time limit work well with attention goals and high-level language goals. They are often paired with cues per set of questions.
    - *"The patient will sustain attention to a simple visual scanning task for 5 minutes with 10 or fewer minimal verbal cues."*
    - *"The patient will participate in complex conversational speech for 10 minutes with 5 or fewer minimal visual cues."*

TYPES OF CUES.
- **Verbal cues.** Verbal instructions for how to produce an accurate response.
- **Visual cues.** Hand gestures and images, like tapping a calendar to remind your patient to use aids to recall the date.
- **Written cues.** Models for writing therapy, written instructions for how to complete a complex task, or written numbers for math problems.
- **Tactile cues.** Touch that helps patients produce an accurate response.
- **Phonemic cues.** Specific sounds during aphasia or motor speech therapy.
- **Articulatory placement cues.** Positioning cues for lips, tongue, and teeth.
- **A mixture of cues** is often helpful. Just remember to record the amount of cueing provided for each type of cue.

REASONABLE. Write short-term goals that are achievable within two weeks. Do this to make sure the goals aren't too challenging and to better measure progress.
- First review your patient's performance on the evaluation.
- For cognitive-communication goals, identify questions where your patient was about 50% accurate. Write goals based on those questions.
    - *For example, if your patient with aphasia answered yes/no questions at 80% accuracy but open-ended questions at 50% accuracy, write a goal for open-ended questions. "The patient will answer auditory open-ended questions at 80% accuracy given moderate written cues."*
- For dysphagia goals, identify the diet level that the patient is currently safe with and write goals for the next advanced diet level (see page 29 for more information about advancing diets) and/or use of safe swallowing strategies.

PRACTICAL. Interview the patient and combine what's reasonable with what's useful and important to the patient.
- Consider your patients' personal goals, what their typical day looks like, how much help they receive with daily tasks, what's important to them, their likes/dislikes, hobbies, and social life.
- Consider **why** you're targeting a goal. Is that **why** practical for your patient?
    - *For example, your patient with dysphagia hates her dentures and hasn't worn them for months, even before her stroke. She prefers soft foods but currently can only safely swallow puréed foods.*
    - *A practical goal would be: "The patient will consume minced & moist textures with appropriate mastication in 90% of opportunities given minimal verbal cues to utilize safe swallowing strategies."*
    - *Her long term goal can include safely swallowing mechanical soft textures, not regular textures, because of her personal preference (hating her dentures!)*

UPGRADE GOALS. Let's say that your patient performs at goal level for 3 sessions in a row. Upgrade a goal by varying different aspects of the goal (e.g., accuracy level, complexity of utterances, etc.)
- Amount and type of cues
- Dysphagia

- Vary liquid textures
- Diet textures
- Presentation: cup sips, self-feeding, etc.
- Amount: teaspoons, 8 oz., entire meal, etc.
- Muscle groups: lingual, oral, pharyngeal, etc.
- Aphasia
    - Vary language comprehension or expression
    - Presentation modality: auditory, visual
    - Response modality: speaking, writing, repetition, etc.
    - Response length: single words, sentences, complex conversations, etc.
    - Response time: such as, "respond within 10 seconds"
- Motor speech
    - Vary response length: phonemes, multisyllabic words, etc.
    - Phoneme and word position: initial, medial, final
    - Presentation modality: auditory, visual
    - Response time
- Voice
    - Quality, pitch, and/or loudness
    - Vary response length: words, phrases, sentences, paragraphs, etc.
    - Response modality: repetition, reading, or talking
- Cognition
    - Vary complexity: simple orientation, complex mathematics, etc.
    - Response time: such as, "complete the puzzle within 5 minutes"
- Visual neglect
    - Vary complexity: reading single words on blank background, searching for specific information on complex map, etc.
    - Response time: such as, "find the target within 2 minutes"

From Aparo & Brewer, 2020

Homework Log

Write down all of your therapy homework (e.g., voice exercises and leg exercises). Next, write down the time you completed each exercise. Get into a routine; try to complete your exercises at the same time everyday.

	HOMEWORK	TIME COMPLETED	NOTES *Effort level, pain, accuracy, questions*
MONDAY			
TUESDAY			
WEDNESDAY			
THURSDAY			
FRIDAY			
SATURDAY			
SUNDAY			

DYSPHAGIA

Dysphagia is difficulty with swallowing. The goal of treatment is to increase the patient's ability to safely consume the least restrictive diet. Choose dysphagia goals and techniques based on what's safe, nutritious, available, possible, what the patient desires, and other relevant factors.

Dysphagia treatment includes:
- Restorative treatment (e.g. swallow strengthening exercises)
- Compensatory treatment (e.g. safe swallowing strategies)

DYSPHAGIA

Page 1 of 4

Therapist Instructions

EVALUATIONS. Complete a case history and bedside swallowing evaluation (include an oral mechanism examination and food and liquid trials).
- The *Mann Assessment of Swallowing Ability* is a good tool for quantifying information collected during the bedside swallowing evaluation (Mann, 2002).
- Many patients will benefit from completing at least one MBSS or FEES. The results of an instrumental evaluation can greatly help when choosing goals, exercises, and strategies. While waiting for results, continue treatment with a focus on providing the safest diet possible (using pertinent strategies and exercises).

DAY ONE OF TREATMENT. Provide the following handouts, as needed.
- Homework Log, Monthly Calendar, Swallowing Impairments, Aspiration Signs & Symptoms, Safe Swallowing, pertinent swallowing exercises, pertinent diet and liquid modification handouts, Incentive Spirometer, Deep Breathing, Directed Cough, Conserve Energy While Eating, Radiation Therapy, Chemotherapy, Tracheostomy Care, Oral Hygiene
- Highlight key points on the handouts, then review with your patients. Ask questions to make sure they understand the content. Answer any questions they may have.

FOR THERAPIST EYES ONLY. Therapist treatment guides are marked with a gray background or header. Some caregivers and patients may benefit from having a copy.
- Cuff Deflation Trials, Neuroplasticity, Dysphagia Devices, Signs of Dysphagia and How to Treat Them, Aspiration Risk Factors, Advancing Diets

SAFE SWALLOWING (PAGE 33). Check off pertinent strategies for each patient. Highlight 2-3 of the most important strategies.
- Review the selected strategies, provide a model, then ask for return demonstrations.
- Every time the patient completes food or liquid trials, have the handout visible and cue your patient to use them.

DYSPHAGIA

SWALLOWING EXERCISES (PAGES 34–47). To treat underlying weakness.
- Copy 2-3 of the most useful exercises. Provide a model then ask for return demonstrations.
- Exercise should be intensive: Have the patient complete these exercises for at least 30 minutes per session with short breaks in between sets.
- Patients should complete exercises daily: Recommend the number of sets for each exercise based on their current level of functioning. 3 sets of 10 repetitions 2 times daily is often recommended.
- Some of the exercises may be interchangeable as they strengthen a similar set of muscles:
  - Mendelsohn Maneuver and Monkey EEE
  - Shaker and Chin Tuck Against Resistance
  - Masako and Hawk

MODIFIED DIETS (PAGES 48–51) & THICKENED LIQUIDS (PAGES 54–55). Review the food items for the patient's recommended diet. Identify foods that the patient will enjoy eating. Help the patient create meal plan ideas. See iddsi.org for more resources *(The International Dysphagia Standardisation Initiative, 2021)*.
- Modify these lists for patients on physician-recommended diets (e.g., renal or diabetic diets).

ESOPHAGEAL (PAGE 52) & HIGH CALORIE DIET (PAGE 53). Handouts for patients whose physicians or dietitians recommend these specific diets.

INCENTIVE SPIROMETER (PAGE 56). Patients may receive an incentive spirometer during an inpatient stay. Provide training, ask for demonstrations, then check in every few days to make sure they're completing this exercise correctly.

DIRECTED COUGH (PAGE 58). For patients who have a weak cough, usually secondary to overall deconditioning or weakness.

DYSPHAGIA

FRAZIER FREE WATER PROTOCOL (PAGE 59).
- Criteria for inclusion: patients who are NPO or on thickened liquids, are able to remain awake and alert while drinking, maintain an upright posture while drinking, have an efficient swallow, and swallow without great discomfort or coughing.
- Patients with **any** of the following should **not** participate in the protocol: unable to consistently get out of bed, have a history of recurrent aspiration pneumonia or acute pulmonary issues, and/or currently have a fever or thrush.

CONSERVE ENERGY WHILE EATING (PAGE 60). For patients who have a history of COPD, heart issues, ALS, or have shortness of breath while seated or with minimal exertion.
- The patient can use a pulse oximeter to monitor oxygen saturation while eating: If below 90%, then consider using energy conservation strategies.

HEAD & NECK CANCER (PAGE 61–63). For use with patients before, during, and after radiation and/or chemotherapy treatment. Patients may also benefit from range of motion exercises and stretches.

TRACHEOSTOMY CARE (PAGE 64) & SPEAKING VALVE (PAGE 67). Review with the caregiver and provide training as appropriate.

ANATOMY & PHYSIOLOGY (PAGE 74–79). Explain anatomy in broad terms, with a focus on the patient's main impairments and how speech therapy can help. See page 553 for an illustration of neck muscles.
- Review swallowing examinations and instrumental evaluations along with the anatomy and physiology handouts.

FACIAL DROOP. Facial paresis can affect chewing, swallowing, and speech. Furthermore, the changes in physical appearance may be psychologically and socially challenging for patients (Konecny et al., 2011).

DYSPHAGIA

- Oral motor exercises are a part of orofacial regulation therapy, mime therapy, and other treatments for facial paresis *(Hagg & Larsson, 2004; Beurskens et al., 2004; Beurskens & Heymans, 2006; Vaughan et al., 2020; Miranda et al., 2015; Santini, n.d.)*
- However, evidence suggests that oral motor exercises must be combined with passive range of motion, active range of motion, massage, biofeedback, and/or facial expression exercises in order to improve facial symmetry or swallowing.
- Refer to PT, OT, oculoplastic surgeons, or maxillofacial surgeons as needed for further treatment options *(Butler & Grobbelaar, 2017)*.

FOOD FOR THOUGHT.
- The best exercise for swallowing is swallowing! Intensity matters, so aim to elicit at least 50 swallows per session.
- Keep in mind that everyone aspirates (even silently) from time to time, so a person who aspirates doesn't necessarily need thickened liquids for a long time.
- Aspiration doesn't automatically mean that a patient will develop pneumonia (see *Aspiration Risk Factors* on page 28).
- Consider your patient's risk factors, cognition, motivation, buy-in, and caregiver support prior to making diet and liquid changes.

DYSPHAGIA

Contents

Cuff Deflation Trials…………………………	20
Speech Trials with Cuff Deflation……………	22
Neuroplasticity……………………………….	24
Dysphagia Devices…………………………	25
Signs of Dysphagia & How to Treat Them…	27
Aspiration Risk Factors……………………..	28
Advancing Diets…………………………….	29
Swallowing Impairments……………………	31
Aspiration Signs & Symptoms………………	32
Safe Swallowing……………………………..	33
Effortful Swallow……………………………..	34
Mendelsohn Maneuver………………………	35
Monkey EEE…………………………………	36
Shaker Exercise…………………………….	37
Chin Tuck Against Resistance………………	38
Super Supraglottic Swallow…………………	39
Masako Maneuver………………………….	40
Hawk…………………………………………	41
Gargle………………………………………..	42
Straw Suck…………………………………..	43
Tongue Press Forward………………………	44
Tongue Press Back…………………………	45
Tongue Press Out……………………………	46
Tongue Press Side………………………….	47
Puréed Diet………………………………….	48
Minced & Moist Diet………………………..	49
Soft & Bite-Sized Diet………………………	50

DYSPHAGIA

Easy to Chew Diet	51
Esophageal Diet	52
High Calorie Diet	53
Thickened Liquids	54
Thickened Liquids Guidelines	55
Incentive Spirometer	56
Deep Breathing	57
Directed Cough	58
Frazier Free Water Protocol	59
Conserve Energy while Eating	60
Head and Neck Stretches	61
Radiation Therapy	62
Chemotherapy	63
Tracheostomy Care	64
Speaking Valve	67
Modified Barium Swallowing Study	69
FEES	71
Oral Hygiene	73
Anatomy and Physiology	74

SEE ALSO

Neuroanatomy & Physiology	189
GERD Tips	554

DYSPHAGIA

Cuff Deflation Trials

Cuff deflation can be scary for our patients, so give plenty of encouragement and education about what you'll be doing during the session and why. For example, explain why you will be touching the pilot balloon prior to reaching for it. Only begin trials if it's been cleared by the physician and/or respiratory therapist and if you've been appropriately trained.

PREPARE THE FOLLOWING SUPPLIES.
- Vital signs monitor
- Clean disposable gloves
- Clean plastic 10 cc syringe
- Watch or timer
- Suctioning catheter
- Tissues (deflating cuffs make some patients cough)
- Oxygen (if the patient uses it continuously or as needed)
- Optional: speaking valve, word lists

CUFF DEFLATION.

1. Position the patient in a comfortable, upright posture. Provide suctioning prior to cuff deflation. Complete tracheostomy care as needed (see page 64).

2. Wash your hands and put on a pair of clean gloves.

3. Monitor the patient's vitals throughout the entire trial. Use a pulse oximeter to monitor their blood oxygen saturation levels. Make sure that saturation levels remain above 90% *(Mayo Clinic Staff, 2018)*. If levels drop below 90%, provide oxygen and try again after saturation stays at normal levels for one minute.

DYSPHAGIA

4. There will be a little pouch (called the "pilot balloon," see page 66 for an illustration) connected to the outside of the trach that is inflated with air when the cuff is inflated. Be prepared to record how many CCs of air you remove from the pouch*.
   - To deflate the cuff, use a clean 10 CC syringe to slowly remove the air in the pouch, about 2 CCs at a time (McKee & Starmer, n.d.) Provide breaks and suctioning as needed.
   - Stop removing air as soon as the pouch is empty of air. You can tell by lightly pinching the pouch; it will feel flat and not bouncy.
   - Record how many CCs of air you removed. This is the same amount you will insert to re-inflate the trach. Place the syringe on a sanitized surface.
   - Continue monitoring the patient's vitals and comfort level.

5. Time how long the patient tolerates cuff deflation.

6. Complete speech trials (page 22) and speaking valve trials (page 67) when the patient is ready to do so.

7. Re-inflate the cuff, inserting the same amount of air that you took out.

8. Continue monitoring the patient's vitals and blood oxygen saturation levels. Leave the room only after their vitals are within normal limits and stable.

9. Communicate with the patient's nurse, physician, and/or respiratory therapist about how the patient tolerated the cuff deflation trial.

*cc=cubic centimeter. 1 cc = 1 mL.

DYSPHAGIA

Speech Trials with Cuff Deflation

Complete the steps on page 20 prior to attempting speech trials. Monitor the patient's vitals throughout the entire trial. Only begin trials if it's been cleared by the physician and/or respiratory therapist and if you've been appropriately trained.

DIGITAL OCCLUSION (BY SLP). Start by placing a clean, gloved finger over the trach during **exhalation only**. Tell the patient that you will cover the trach while they exhale so that they can produce a voice.

SIMPLE PHONATION. Start with vowel sounds, "hello," or their name.
- Ask the patient to take a deep breath. Immediately after inhalation, provide digital occlusion and ask them to speak. Make sure to **release your finger immediately after they speak** so that the patient can inhale.
- The patient typically requires at least a few attempts before producing any voice. Give the patient a short break (a few breaths) between each trial. Provide plenty of encouragement.
- Continue to monitor the patient's vitals.

DIGITAL OCCLUSION (BY PATIENT). Once the patient feels comfortable, they may provide the digital occlusion. Make sure that they are using a clean, gloved finger.
- Start by asking the patient to simply practice occlusion by taking a deep breath then saying a vowel sound during occlusion.
- The patient may also practice coughing and throat clearing during digital occlusion.

CHECK O2 SATURATION. Carefully monitor the patient's vitals and fatigue levels. The first couple of trials may only last a few minutes. Again, give plenty of encouragement.

DYSPHAGIA

RE-INFLATE THE CUFF (AS APPLICABLE). When trials are completed, re-inflate the cuff by placing the clean syringe back into the pilot balloon and inserting the same amount of air (in CCs) that you removed prior to speech trials *(McKee & Starmer, n.d.)* Ensure that the patient's vitals remain stable before leaving the patient alone.

INCREASE THE CHALLENGE. Gradually work your way up to several minutes of deflation with speech trials. You may eventually use a one-way speaking valve (e.g. *Passy Muir®* Valve, see page 67) to produce a voice instead of digital occlusion.

INTERDISCIPLINARY CARE. Keep the patient's physician and/or respiratory therapist in the loop by providing weekly (or more frequent) updates on how speech trials are progressing.
- Discuss your recommendations and ask whether it's medically safe to continue with your plan of care (e.g., using a speaking valve, encouraging cuff deflation for longer periods of time, etc.)
- Once you have this medical clearance, gradually work your way up to an hour, several hours, and day-long deflations.
- Train the patient and caregivers on how to properly deflate and re-inflate the cuff. Encourage the patient to obtain a pulse oximeter to monitor oxygen saturation throughout the day.

DYSPHAGIA

Neuroplasticity

Neuroplasticity is the brain's ability to reorganize and make new connections in response to experience or after an injury. Take advantage of neuroplasticity to enhance your treatments (Robbins et al., 2008; Kleim & Jones, 2008).

USE IT OR LOSE IT. Function can be lost if the associated part of the brain isn't activated.

USE IT AND IMPROVE IT. "Practice makes perfect."

SPECIFICITY. The brain will reorganize and make new connections in the parts of the brain that are being used during an action.

REPETITION. Repeat an action often and over an extended period of time. Behavioral changes occur before brain changes do.

INTENSITY. A certain threshold (e.g., length of exercise, number of sessions) must be reached in order to induce neuroplasticity.

TIME. Sustained practice can maximize neuroplasticity.

SALIENCE. The function must be meaningful to the patient to maximize plasticity.

AGE. Although younger brains have more neuroplasticity, older brains can still change, although at a slower rate.

TRANSFERENCE. Neuroplasticity from one training experience (e.g. loud speech) can sometimes "transfer" to, or enhance, related skills (swallowing).

INTERFERENCE. Not all neuroplasticity is desirable. An example is a compensatory behavior that interferes with learning the desired function.

Dysphagia Devices

The following dysphagia devices may strengthen chewing and swallowing musculature and/or reduce the signs and symptoms of dysphagia. Inexpensive and easily accessible treatments are described later in this chapter.

IOPI®. *The Iowa Oral Performance Instrument* is used to increase and measure lip and tongue strength (Robbins et al., 2007). It features an air-filled bulb on one end and a hand-held measurement device on the other. It provides visual biofeedback in the form of a row of lights.

sEMG. Surface electromyography uses electrodes placed on the skin of the lower face and/or neck to measure muscle activity. sEMG provides visual biofeedback via a row of lights or a graph on a computer screen. sEMG is especially helpful for training in the Mendelsohn maneuver and effortful swallow. There are many sEMG manufacturers and models, including the *Pathway® MR* series by The Prometheus Group.

EMST. Expiratory Muscle Strength Training strengthens expiratory and submental muscles which are important when breathing out forcefully, swallowing, and coughing. Patients blow strong and fast into the *EMST150™* device until they reach a specified threshold of pressure. EMST has been shown to improve suprahyoid movement and penetration-aspiration scale scores (Park et al., 2016).

ORAL SCREENS. These are orthodontic devices that look similar to a mouth guard with a plastic ring on the outside. They may help with lip strengthening (Hagg & Anniko, 2008). Oral screens are typically custom fit by orthodontists. The *Muppy®* by Dr. Hinz Dental is an inexpensive oral screen.

DYSPHAGIA

NMES. Neuromuscular electrical stimulation delivers small electrical currents via electrodes placed on the skin of the face and/or neck. The current causes muscles to contract, which can help during swallowing exercises *(Tan et al., 2013)*. *VitalStim®* is an NMES device that has been approved by the FDA.

CPAP. A continuous positive airway pressure machine is often prescribed by physicians to treat obstructive sleep apnea. CPAP is also used to improve hypernasal resonance *(Kuehn, 1991)*, and there's emerging evidence that it can reduce premature spillage for people with obstructive sleep apnea *(Caparroz et al., 2019)*.

DYSPHAGIA

Signs of Dysphagia & How to Treat Them

Anterior spillage	thickened liquids, small bites and sips, labial exercises
Inadequate mastication	modified diet textures, small bites and sips, lingual exercises
Uncoordinated oral phase	bolus hold, lingual exercises, small bites and sips
Oral residue	alternating bites and sips, lingual sweep, lingual exercises
Pharyngeal pooling	thickened liquids, small bites and sips, bolus hold, chin tuck, lingual exercises
Nasal regurgitation	small bites and sips, thinner consistencies, Masako maneuver, Hawk, Mendelsohn maneuver, Monkey EEE, Shaker exercise, Chin Tuck Against Resistance
Reduced epiglottic movement	Mendelsohn maneuver, Monkey EEE, effortful swallow
Vallecular residue	dry swallow, alternating bites and sips, effortful swallow, Mendelsohn maneuver, Monkey EEE, lingual exercises
Reduced UES opening	head turn, Mendelsohn maneuver, Monkey EEE, Shaker exercise, Chin Tuck Against Resistance
Pyriform sinus residue	dry swallow, alternating bites and sips, head turn, Mendelsohn maneuver, Monkey EEE, Shaker exercise, Chin Tuck Against Resistance
Laryngeal penetration	thickened liquids, small bites and sips, alternating bites and sips, bolus hold, chin tuck, Mendelsohn maneuver, Monkey EEE, effortful swallow

The Adult Speech Therapy Workbook © 2021 Chung Hwa Brewer

DYSPHAGIA

Aspiration Risk Factors

The following conditions put your patients at higher risk for aspiration.

- Poor oral hygiene or dentition
- Reduced saliva—often related to Sjogren's syndrome or history of radiation and chemotherapy for head and neck cancer *(Cedars-Sinai, 2021)*
- Dysphonia
- Dysarthria
- Abnormal or weak cough
- Needing help with feeding or oral care *(Langmore et al., 1998)*
- Resisting feeding
- History of smoking
- Feeling full very quickly
- Weight loss
- Dehydration
- Taking extra effort/time to complete meals
- History of respiratory infections/pneumonia
- Taking multiple swallows every bite or sip
- Acid reflux
- Tongue pumping
- Impulsive eating behaviors

DYSPHAGIA

Advancing Diets

For patients who are on modified diets.

FACTORS TO CONSIDER. How quickly you advance textures will depend on the patient's physical and cognitive functioning and on the physician's orders.
- **Physical functioning.** Ability to sit upright, feed self, produce a strong cough, move neck, chew and swallow, fatigue level, current respiratory functioning (e.g., acute or recurrent aspiration pneumonia, COPD, heart failure, etc.), pain level, cancer status (e.g., post lingual resection, currently receiving radiation, etc.), etc.
- **Cognitive functioning.** Ability to stay awake, attend to food, control impulses, recall swallowing strategies, type and severity of neurological impairment (e.g., brainstem stroke, ALS, etc.), etc.

YOUR PATIENT'S FIRST MODIFIED DIET. In most cases, this diet will be the textures that the patient safely consumes in 80% or more of opportunities.
- Complete an instrumental evaluation, oral mechanism examination, and bedside swallowing evaluation.
- An NPO diet is appropriate for patients who have no swallowing reflex or no UES opening *(Richard, 2017)*. It's not appropriate for all patients that aspirate; consider that even on an NPO diet, a patient can aspirate on saliva or reflux content.

FOOD & LIQUID TRIALS.
- If the patient is **alert and oriented**, begin by trialing small amounts of the previous level of function (PLOF) diet.
    - For example, teaspoon of thin liquids and teaspoon of regular textures.
    - If they tolerate small amounts well, trial larger amounts (e.g., cup sips of thin liquids and normal-sized bites of regular textures).
- If the patient has a **hard time staying awake**, attempt trials when the patient is more alert. Ask a caregiver, nurse, or their other therapists what times the patient is typically more alert.

DYSPHAGIA

ADD SAFE SWALLOWING STRATEGIES. If the patient demonstrates some signs or symptoms of dysphagia during the food and liquid trials, introduce safe swallowing strategies. Complete a few more food and liquid trials using the strategies and observe whether those signs or symptoms improve.
- If the strategies consistently improve the signs or symptoms AND the patient safely consumes the food and liquids in 80-100% of trials: Your dysphagia goal would be to continue trials with a speech therapist using those strategies.
    - You may upgrade to these textures once they've demonstrated safe swallowing AND consistent use of strategies across three sessions.
- If the patient still demonstrates the same signs or symptoms of dysphagia, then trial thicker liquids and/or softer foods. Add in safe swallowing strategies with these textures.
    - Modify the diet until the patient safely consumes the food and liquids in 80-100% of trials while using the strategies.

ADD SWALLOWING EXERCISES. Use exercises to improve underlying weakness or discoordination. Add pertinent swallowing exercises to your patient's modified diet and safe swallowing strategies.
- Exercises should be intensive with a high number of repetitions.

FOLLOW-UP INSTRUMENTAL EVALUATIONS. Recommend repeat MBSS and FEES as appropriate. Patients with severe pharyngeal dysphagia may need 3 or more instrumental evaluations throughout their time in speech therapy.

GETTING OFF AN NPO DIET. Many patients who are NPO and/or receive tube feedings can recover enough to resume a fully PO diet. Communicate regularly with the patient's physician, dietician, gastroenterologist, and/or respiratory therapist to ensure that the patient is safe and receives adequate nutrition for a PO diet.
- Get physician clearance that the patient is medically stable enough to begin PO trials.
- Complete an instrumental evaluation and swallowing mechanism evaluation to determine appropriate PO textures, swallowing strategies, and exercises to trial.
- Complete food and liquid trials as described above.
- Monitor vitals, fatigue level, and lung sounds each session.

DYSPHAGIA

Swallowing Impairments

Common impairments related to dysphagia include:

ORAL DYSPHAGIA. Difficulties with feeding and chewing.

PHARYNGEAL DYSPHAGIA. Difficulties with swallowing.

OROPHARYNGEAL DYSPHAGIA. Difficulties with chewing and swallowing.

PHARYNGOESOPHAGEAL DYSPHAGIA. Difficulties with swallowing at the throat and esophagus levels.

ESOPHAGEAL DYSPHAGIA. Difficulties with swallowing from the esophagus downward.

LARYNGEAL PENETRATION. Food or liquid going towards the airway.

ASPIRATION. Food or liquid entering the airway.

ASPIRATION PNEUMONIA. Lung infection caused by inhaling food or liquid.

DYSPHAGIA

Aspiration Signs & Symptoms

Aspiration is when food or liquid enters the airway. It can cause serious medical issues, including pneumonia.

- Coughing after eating or drinking
- Clearing your throat after eating or drinking
- Wet or gurgly sounding voice after eating or drinking
- Recurrent sore throat
- Feeling that food is stuck in your throat after swallowing
- Chest congestion
- Difficulty breathing
- Shortness of breath
- Fever starting 30-60 minutes after eating *(Cedars-Sinai, 2021)*

DYSPHAGIA

Safe Swallowing

Only complete the strategies that your therapist checked off.

- ☐ Take a sip of your drink, look down at your lap, then swallow. *(Saconato, 2016)*
- ☐ After each swallow, clear your throat and swallow again.
- ☐ Hold each bite/sip in your mouth for 3 seconds, then swallow.
- ☐ After each bite of food, take a sip of your drink.
- ☐ Take small bites, one at a time. *(Stevens, 2011)*
- ☐ After each bite, set your utensil down and eat slowly.
- ☐ Swallow each bite/sip **twice**.
- ☐ After each bite/sip, turn your head and then swallow.
- ☐ Sit bolt upright whenever you eat or drink. *(Sura et al., 2012)*
- ☐ Sit upright for at least 30 minutes after eating.
- ☐ Use a teaspoon or a small fork.
- ☐ Swallow **hard** like you're swallowing a whole grape.
- ☐ Use your tongue to clear out any leftovers in your mouth.
- ☐ Avoid straws and drink straight from the cup.
- ☐ Use straws to avoid tilting your head back when you drink.
- ☐ Place your medications in apple sauce, yogurt, or pudding.
- ☐ Cut your pills in half.
- ☐ Crush your pills and place them in apple sauce, yogurt, or pudding.
- ☐ Avoid speaking while there's food in your mouth.
- ☐ Eat only when you feel awake and alert.
- ☐ Reduce distractions while you eat. Do not watch TV or read.

DYSPHAGIA

Effortful Swallow

This exercise is meant increase pressure in your mouth, throat, and esophagus (Huckabee & Steele, 2006).

---

1. Swallow **as hard as you can** (pretend that you're swallowing a whole grape).
2. Repeat 10 times.

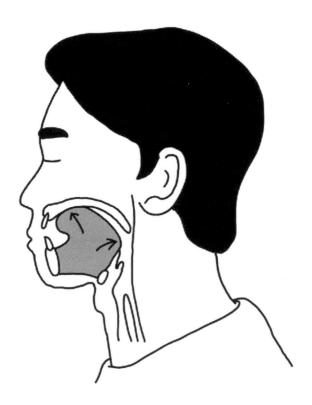

DYSPHAGIA

Mendelsohn Maneuver

This exercise is meant to elevate the voice box and open the esophagus (Boden et al., 2006).

---

1. Swallow your saliva and feel your Adam's apple move up and down.
2. Place your tongue tip against the ridge that's behind your front teeth.
3. Swallow your saliva again, but halfway through the swallow, hold your Adam's apple up using the muscles under your chin.
4. **Hold** it up for 1-3 seconds.
5. Repeat 10 times.

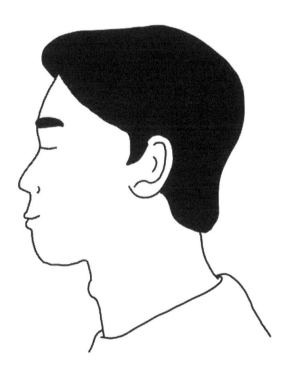
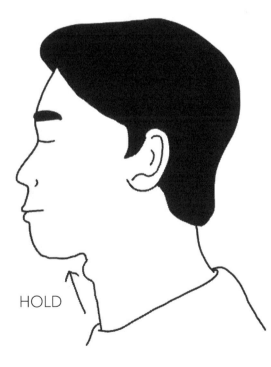

HOLD

> **DYSPHAGIA**

Monkey EEE

Also known as "effortful pitch glide." This exercise is meant to lift the voice box (Miloro et al., 2014).

---

1. Say "eee" in your normal voice.
2. Continue saying "eee" as you quickly glide up to your **highest pitch** possible.
3. Continue saying "eee" as you **apply force** to make a strong "eee" sound.
4. Take a breath.
5. Repeat 10 times.

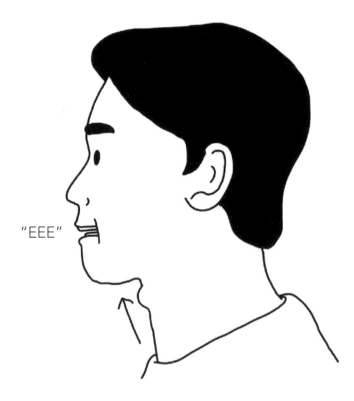

DYSPHAGIA

Shaker Exercise

Pronounced "sha-KEER," this exercise is meant to help open the sphincter at the top of your esophagus (Shaker et al., 1997).

---

1. Lay flat on your back, do not use a pillow.
2. Raise your head to look at your toes (keep your shoulders on the ground) and hold for up to 60 seconds.
   - Breathe through your nose.
3. Relax back down for 60 seconds.
4. Complete two more times.
5. **Next**, raise your head and hold up for 3 seconds. Relax down.
6. Repeat the 3-second hold (relaxing down between each repetition) up to 30 times.

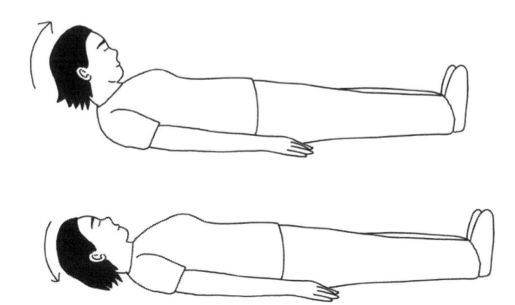

> DYSPHAGIA

Chin Tuck Against Resistance

This exercise is meant to strengthen the muscles under the chin (Yoon et al., 2014).

---

1. While seated, place a rolled-up hand towel under your chin, pressed lightly against your neck.
    - You may also place a squishy ball or your fist under your chin.
2. Press your chin down into the towel and hold down for 60 seconds.
    - Keep your spine straight.
3. Relax for 60 seconds. Complete two more times.
4. **Next**, press your chin down into the towel and hold for 3 seconds.
5. Relax then repeat the 3-second hold (relaxing between each repetition) up to 30 times.

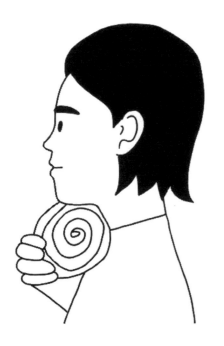 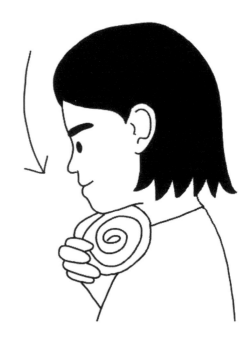

DYSPHAGIA

Super Supraglottic Swallow

This technique is meant to close off the airway before and during a swallow. This reduces the risk for aspiration (Donzelli & Brady, 2004).

---

1. Take a deep breath and hold it in **tight**.
2. Take a bite or a sip. Continue to hold your breath.
3. Swallow hard.
4. Immediately after swallowing, **cough**.
5. Breathe.

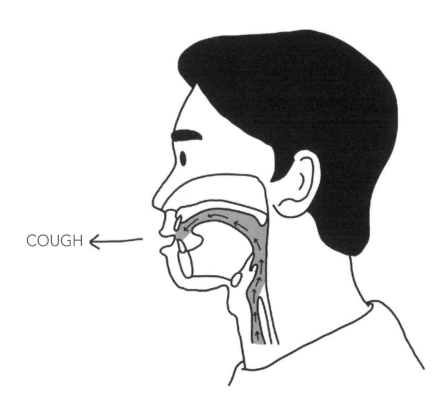

DYSPHAGIA

Masako Maneuver

This exercise strengthens the back wall of the throat (Fujiu & Logemann, 1996).

---

1. Stick your tongue out and hold it gently between your lips.
   - Relax your eyes and cheeks.
2. Swallow and keep sticking your tongue out.
3. Repeat 10 times.

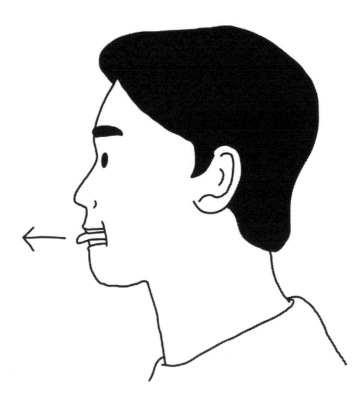

DYSPHAGIA

Hawk

This exercise improves movement of the back wall of the throat (Perlman et al., 1989).

---

1. Say the word "hawk" in a loud voice, emphasizing the "k" sound.
   - It will sound like "haw-KKH."
2. Repeat 10 times.

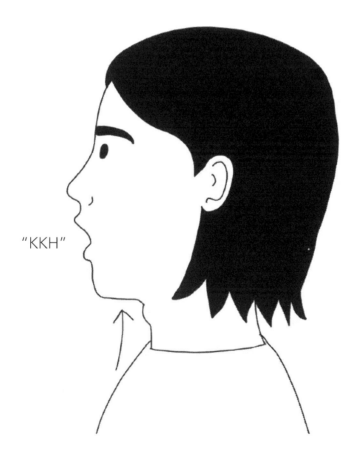

DYSPHAGIA

Gargle

Use this technique to improve movement of the back of your tongue (Provencio-Arambula et al., 2007).

---

1. Pretend to gargle for 5 seconds.
2. Repeat 10 times.

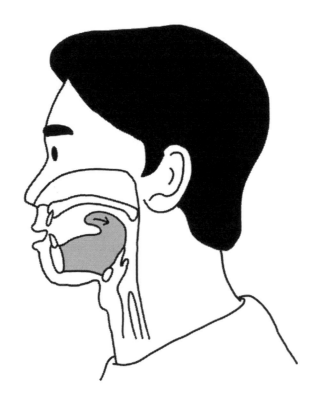

DYSPHAGIA

Straw Suck

This exercise is meant to strengthen your lips (Richard, 2017; Dysphagia Ramblings, 2019).

---

1. Place your lips around a straw (regular size or cocktail size).
2. Place the straw in a thickened liquid (e.g., honey thick or pudding thick).
3. Suck continuously for 3 seconds or until the liquid reaches your mouth.
   - If the liquid reaches your mouth, swallow it **hard**.
4. Pause, then repeat for a total of 10 sucks.

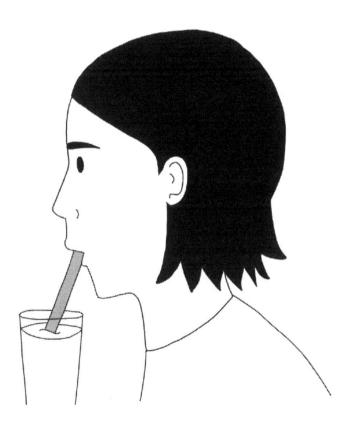

DYSPHAGIA

Tongue Press Forward

This exercise strengthens the tongue (McKenna et al., 2017).

---

1. Lift the front part of your tongue (more than just the tongue tip).
2. Press it against the ridge that's behind your top front teeth.
3. Hold and press for 10 seconds.
4. Relax. Repeat 10 times.

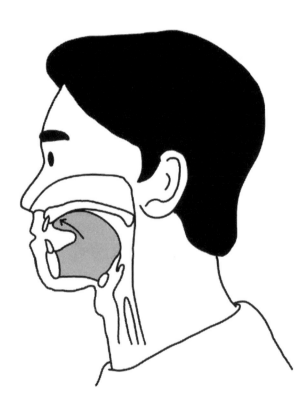

DYSPHAGIA

Tongue Press Back

This exercise strengthens the tongue (Namiki et al., 2019).

---

1. Lift the back of your tongue.
2. Press it against the hard palate, right before it meets the soft palate.
3. Hold and press for 10 seconds.
4. Relax. Repeat 10 times.

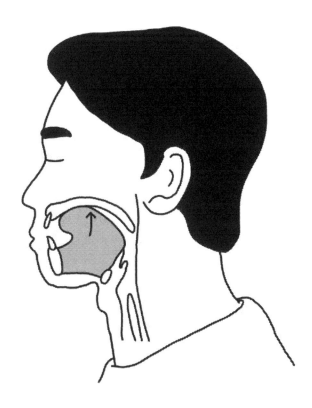

DYSPHAGIA

Tongue Press Out

This exercise strengthens the tongue (Clark et al., 2009).

---

1. Gently bite down on a tongue depressor placed between your upper and lower front teeth.
2. Press your tongue against the tongue depressor.
    - You may hold the tongue depressor in place with your hand if it shifts.
3. Continue pressing for 10 seconds.
    - Remember to **gently** bite down on the tongue depressor.
4. Pause and repeat for a total of 10 presses.

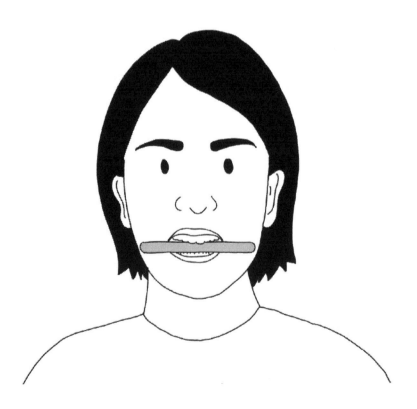

DYSPHAGIA

Tongue Press Side

This exercise strengthens the tongue (Clark et al., 2009).

---

1. Gently bite down on a tongue depressor placed between your upper and lower premolars.
2. Press the side of your tongue against the tongue depressor.
   - You may hold the tongue depressor in place with your hand if it shifts.
3. Continue pressing for 10 seconds.
   - Remember to **gently** bite down on the tongue depressor.
4. Pause and repeat for a total of 10 presses.
5. Switch sides and repeat steps 1-5.

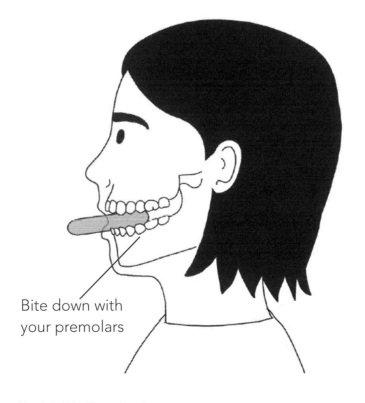

Bite down with your premolars

> DYSPHAGIA

Puréed Diet

Also known as "Blended" diet. You shouldn't have to chew. Food should be smooth and moist with no chunks (Maryland Department of Health and Mental Hygiene, 2014).

Avoid *crunchy or crumbly foods (chips, popcorn, nuts), seeds, rice, stringy vegetables (green beans), and vegetables and fruit with skins (potatoes, peaches, grapes).*

RECOMMENDED FOODS.
- Puréed cottage cheese
- Pudding, custard, *Magic Cup®* ice cream
- Thickened smoothies (remove seeds)
- Puréed meat including beef, pork, poultry, fish, and shellfish
- Soft tofu
- Puréed cooked vegetables
- Mashed potatoes (no skin)
- Mashed canned fruit (remove fruit skin and seeds)
- Apple sauce
- Mashed bananas
- Cream of wheat
- Blended oatmeal
- Puréed soup (including tomato soup)
- Butter, gravy, ketchup, honey, syrup

DYSPHAGIA

Minced & Moist Diet

Also known as "Ground," "Dysphagia Mechanical," or "Mechanically Altered" diet. Your food should be moist and minced (Maryland Department of Health and Mental Hygiene, 2014).

Avoid *bread, crunchy or crumbly foods (chips, popcorn, nuts), seeds, stringy vegetables (green beans), and vegetables or fruit with skins (grapes, potatoes, peaches).*

RECOMMENDED FOODS.
- All foods in the puréed diet
- Very soft ground meat including beef and poultry
- Tofu
- Ripe avocados
- Tuna salad and egg salad (no relish, pickles, or nuts)
- Soft cooked eggs
- Soft cooked vegetables
- Soft bananas
- Soft, well cooked pasta
- Cream soups (no large vegetable chunks or noodles)
- Rice pudding

DYSPHAGIA

Soft & Bite-Sized Diet

Also known as "Mechanical Soft," "Diced," or "Chopped" diet. Your food should be soft and moist and pieces should be bite-sized (Maryland Department of Health and Mental Hygiene, 2014).

Avoid *dry or tough meats (bacon, hot dogs, sausages), dried fruit, bread with hard crusts, seeds, nuts, and hard or chewy candy.*

RECOMMENDED FOODS.
- All foods in the minced & moist and puréed diets
- Cheese
- Diced meat
- Canned beans
- Moist meatballs
- Soft-cooked, boneless fish
- Casseroles with tender meat and vegetables
- Eggs
- Soft-cooked potatoes
- Canned green beans
- Canned fruit
- Soft pancakes and French toast
- Simple dry cereals with milk (no hard-to-chew cereals, like granola)
- Cake, soft cookies, and pie (without crunchy pieces)

DYSPHAGIA

Easy to Chew Diet

Also known as "Dysphagia Advanced," "Advanced Soft," or "Dental" diet.

Avoid *tough, dry, or crunchy foods like steak, toast, or granola* (Maryland Department of Health and Mental Hygiene, 2014).

RECOMMENDED FOODS.
- All foods in the soft & bite-sized, minced & moist, and puréed diets
- Peanut butter
- Shredded lettuce
- Berries
- Creamed corn
- Legumes
- Soft ripe peaches, nectarines, kiwis, cantaloupe, honeydew, seedless watermelon, etc.
- Bread, biscuits, muffins, pancakes, French toast, and waffles
- Tortillas
- Cereal moistened with milk
- Rice
- Corn chowder and clam chowder

DYSPHAGIA

Esophageal Diet

This diet is for people with a history of esophageal strictures or esophageal dilation (Brunt et al., n.d.)

Avoid *alcohol, fibrous meat (steak, bacon, sausage), chunky peanut butter, bread, popcorn, rice, raw vegetables, lettuce, nuts, seeds, dry fruit, and chips* (hoag.org, 2012).

RECOMMENDED FOODS.
- Cream of wheat, oatmeal, cornflakes softened with milk
- Jell-O, pudding, custard
- Baked, canned, and cooked fruit
- Ripe bananas, skinless peaches, skinless nectarines, and skinless pears
- Soft tender beef, chicken, and boneless fish
- Eggs
- Cooked beans
- Casseroles with ground meat
- Smooth peanut butter
- Cottage cheese
- Baked and mashed potatoes (skin removed)
- Soft cookies
- Soft pasta
- Cream soups
- Canned or cooked vegetables without seeds or skins
- Ripe avocados
- Yogurt without fruit
- Gravy

DYSPHAGIA

High Calorie Diet

Try adding the following foods to your diet if you take a long time finishing meals or you continually lose weight. These foods can help you gain weight or avoid further weight loss. Consider visiting a nutritionist or dietitian for more information.

- **Avocados** (Mawer, 2020)
- Eggs
- Tofu
- Beans
- Protein shakes
- Whole milk
- Whole milk cheese, yogurt, cottage cheese, and sour cream
- Potatoes
- Squash
- Soft corn
- Salmon
- Soft rice with cheese sauce
- Pasta
- Peanut butter
- Other nut butters
- Butter or margarine
- Mayonnaise
- Salad dressing
- Extra virgin olive oil, avocado oil, and coconut oil

DYSPHAGIA

Thickened Liquids

You can buy thickeners at major retailers. Common brands are Resource Thicken Up®, Hormel Thick & Easy®, and Thick-It®. These thickeners use xantham gum. They remain stable over time and in varied temperatures (Mills, 2008). In contrast, starch-based thickeners aren't as stable, so are often not recommended.

THIN LIQUIDS. Most drinks, including water, coffee, and milk.

SLIGHTLY THICK. Also known as "natural nectar thick." These liquids are between thin and mildly thick consistencies. Includes drinks like apricot juice and tomato juice.

MILDLY THICK. Also known as "nectar thick." Similar to the consistency of thick chocolate milk or creamy soup (Maryland Department of Health and Mental Hygiene, 2014).

EXTREMELY THICK. Also known as "honey thick." Similar to the consistency of honey. These liquids can be poured, but they move slowly when shaken.

LIQUIDS IN FOODS. Avoid foods that melt, like ice cream and smoothies, and are very juicy, like oranges or melons. Drain canned fruits and vegetables before eating them.

DYSPHAGIA

Thickened Liquids Guidelines

LIQUIDS THAT SHOULD BE THICKENED:

- Water
- Coffee and Tea
- Milk
- Soda
- Juice and vegetable juice
- Nutritional shakes
- Broth
- Soup
- Etc.

AVOID FOODS THAT MELT.

- No ice cubes
- No jello
- No ice cream, frozen yogurt, Italian ice, popsicles, and sherbet
- No smoothies
- No milkshakes and malts
- No hard candy
- No cough drops

> DYSPHAGIA

Incentive Spirometer

Incentive spirometers improve lung health and help you take slow, deep breaths (MedlinePlus, 2019). *This is important when recovering from certain lung illnesses and surgeries. Continue using the spirometer for as long as your doctor or therapist recommends.*

---

1. Breathe out normally, then place the mouthpiece between your lips.
2. **Breathe in** deeply through your mouth.
    - Watch the flow rate guide (usually a blue disc) rise up to the goal level.
3. Continue breathing in for as long as you can (or as long your doctor, therapist, or nurse instructed).
4. Breathe out slowly and relax.
5. After 10 repetitions, cough.

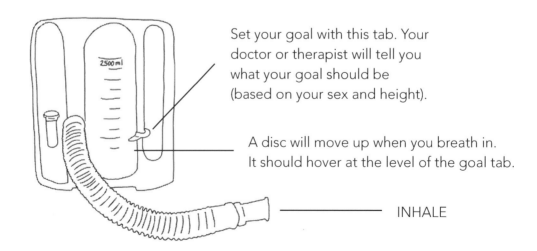

Set your goal with this tab. Your doctor or therapist will tell you what your goal should be (based on your sex and height).

A disc will move up when you breath in. It should hover at the level of the goal tab.

INHALE

DYSPHAGIA

Deep Breathing

Deep breathing is also called "diaphragmatic breathing." It helps you breathe from the diaphragm instead of your throat or shoulders (Jewell, 2018). This helps you take deeper breaths. See page 449 for a side view of the lungs and stomach.

---

1. Place one hand on your stomach and one hand on your chest.
2. Breathe in deeply through your nose.
   - Push out your stomach when you inhale. Your chest should remain still.
3. Exhale slowly through your mouth.
   - Feel your stomach pull in. Your chest should remain still.
4. Repeat steps 2-3 for a few minutes.

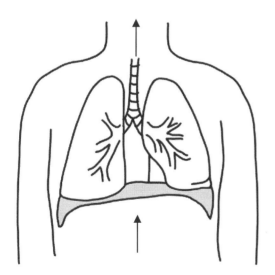

EXHALATION. The diaphragm is shaded in gray.

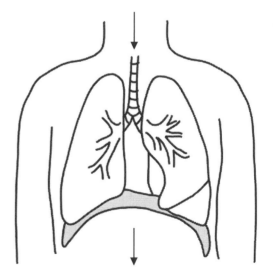

INHALATION. The lungs expand and the diaphragm contracts down.

DYSPHAGIA

Directed Cough

Follow these steps to produce a stronger cough. This can help get out any "junk" that may have settled in your lungs.

---

1. Sit up straight.
2. Take a deep breath, hold for a second.
3. Squeeze your abdominal muscles to cough **big**.
4. Relax and breathe.
5. Repeat as needed.

DYSPHAGIA

Frazier Free Water Protocol

This protocol allows people who meet specific qualifying criteria to drink un-thickened water. It helps them stay hydrated while decreasing their risk for aspiration (Panther, 2005). Water has a neutral pH and low bacteria count compared to saliva. If your mouth, teeth, and tongue are clean, it is less likely that the water you drink will carry bacteria into your lungs if you aspirate.

WHO QUALIFIES. You must meet **all** of the following qualifications:
- NPO or on thickened liquids
- Alert and upright posture while drinking.
- Get out of bed consistently.
- Have an efficient swallow without great discomfort or coughing.
- **No** history of recurrent aspiration pneumonia or acute pulmonary issues.
- **No** current fever or thrush.

YOU MUST COMPLETE THE FOLLOWING.
- Brush your teeth and tongue 2-3 times daily.
- **Do not** drink unthickened water while eating. Only drink thickened liquids while eating.
- You must **wait 30 minutes after eating** to drink unthickened water.
- Water is given only when you request it. You will get one cup of water at a time versus a large water bottle.
- Do not take medications with water. Add medications to applesauce, yogurt, or pudding.
- Use swallowing strategies as needed while drinking water.

DYSPHAGIA

Conserve Energy while Eating

If you have shortness of breath or fatigue easily, eating may be challenging or uncomfortable (Tabor et al., 2017). *Use these strategies to increase safety and to feel more comfortable while eating.*

- Eat only when you're fully awake and alert.
- Reduce distractions while you're eating: turn off the TV, don't read a book or magazine, etc.
- Avoid speaking with food in your mouth.
- Eat softer foods and avoid tough foods that require a lot of chewing.
- Take small bites and sips (Healthwise Staff, 2020).
- Use smaller utensils to reduce the size of each bite.
- Take only one bite or sip at a time.
- Place your eating utensils down between bites.
- Take small breaks throughout your meal.
- Sit upright during and for 30 minutes after the meal.
- Eat higher calorie foods that are healthy (e.g. avocado, whole milk yogurt, cheese, peanut butter) if your physician-recommended diet allows for it.

DYSPHAGIA

Head and Neck Stretches

Sit in a straight-backed chair (e.g. dining chair—not a sofa or recliner) and breathe deeply. Slowly inhale then exhale for a few breaths. Remember your slow breathing as you stretch. Hold each stretch for about one minute (Freutel, 2020).

---

1. Slowly roll your shoulders back, keeping your neck and jaw relaxed.
   - Your mouth may hang open a little bit and that's okay.
2. Slowly roll your shoulder forward, keeping your neck and jaw relaxed.
3. Lean your head to one side and relax, slowing sinking your ear toward your shoulder with every slow breath.
4. Lean your head to the other side, slowly sinking your ear toward your shoulder with every breath.
   - Continue to relax and breathe slowly. Relax you neck and jaw.
5. Slowly roll your neck forward from side to side.
6. Slowly roll your neck back from side to side.
7. Turn you head as if looking over your shoulder.
   - Keep your shoulders and jaw relaxed.
8. Switch sides and look over your other shoulder.

DYSPHAGIA

Radiation Therapy

Speech therapy before and during radiation therapy for head or neck cancer can significantly decrease some of the negative side effects of radiation.

COMMON SIDE EFFECTS.
- Skin dryness, itching, blistering, or peeling *(Memorial Sloan Kettering Cancer Center, 2018)*
- Dry mouth
- Mouth sores
- Mouth pain
- Difficulty swallowing
- Jaw stiffness
- Nausea
- Hair loss
- Tooth decay
- Thick saliva
- Taste changes
- Hoarse voice
- Fatigue
- Reduced muscle range of motion

WHAT YOU CAN DO.
- Brush your teeth twice a day
- Floss before you go to bed
- Rinse your mouth with water or mouthwash (non-alcohol) every 4-6 hours
- Use chapstick
- Use a humidifier
- Use skin moisturizer
- Use products like *Biotène®* mouth spray, toothpaste, or mouthwash to help with dry mouth
- Do your chewing and swallowing exercises to maintain muscle strength and range of motion (speak to your speech therapist for more details)

DYSPHAGIA

Chemotherapy

Speech therapy before and during chemotherapy for head and neck cancer can significantly decrease some of the negative side effects of chemotherapy.

COMMON SIDE EFFECTS.
- Taste changes *(National Cancer Institute, 2019)*
- Dry mouth
- Pain
- Bleeding easily in the mouth
- Tooth decay and gum disease
- Nerve damage
- Reduced muscle range of motion

WHAT YOU CAN DO.
- Brush your teeth twice a day
- Floss before you go to bed
- Rinse your mouth with water or mouthwash (non-alcohol) every 4-6 hours
- Use chapstick
- Use a humidifier
- Use products like Biotène mouth spray, toothpaste, or mouthwash to help with dry mouth
- Do your chewing and swallowing exercises to maintain muscle strength and range of motion (speak to your speech therapist for more details)

DYSPHAGIA

Tracheostomy Care

Complete tracheostomy care only after you have been properly trained by a nurse or therapist. Position the patient in an upright posture. Monitor the patient's vitals and oxygen saturation levels with a pulse oximeter when handling their tracheostomy.

SUPPLIES YOU WILL NEED.
- Clean disposable gloves
- Suction and catheter (usually a Yankauer)
- Hydrogen peroxide
- Clean gauze
- Sterile water
- Clean dry towels or paper towels
- Small clean brush or pipe cleaners
- Four clean bowls
- Pulse oximeter

(John Hopkins Medicine, n.d.-a)

WHAT TO DO.
1. Position the patient in a comfortable, upright posture.
2. Wash your hands with antibacterial soap, dry them with paper towels or an electric hand dryer, then put on a pair of clean gloves.
3. Clean the suction catheter prior to suctioning the trach:

DYSPHAGIA

- Place some hydrogen peroxide in a bowl and suction it up using the suction catheter until all mucus inside the catheter is washed away.
- Wipe the catheter with a clean piece of gauze.
- In the second clean bowl, add some sterile water. Suction the water with the suction catheter until all the hydrogen peroxide is washed away.
- Suction air until the catheter is dry on the inside.
- Remove catheter from tubing and let air dry.

4. Wash and dry your hands again then put on a new pair of clean gloves.
5. Place a solution of 1/2 sterile water and 1/2 hydrogen peroxide in the third clean bowl, and sterile water only in the fourth clean bowl.
6. Remove the inner cannula of the trach while holding onto the neck plate*.
7. Place the inner cannula in the hydrogen peroxide solution until any hardened matter softens.
8. Use a brush or pipe cleaners to clean the inside and outside of the inner cannula.
9. Rinse the cannula in sterile water and dry with a clean, dry towel.
10. Reinsert the inner cannula into the trach while holding the neck plate, turning the cannula until it locks into position.

While cleaning the inner cannula, the patient continues to breathe through the trach. If the patient requires oxygen, then the oxygen mask can still be placed over the trach. Remember to clean or replace the mask, as appropriate.

DYSPHAGIA

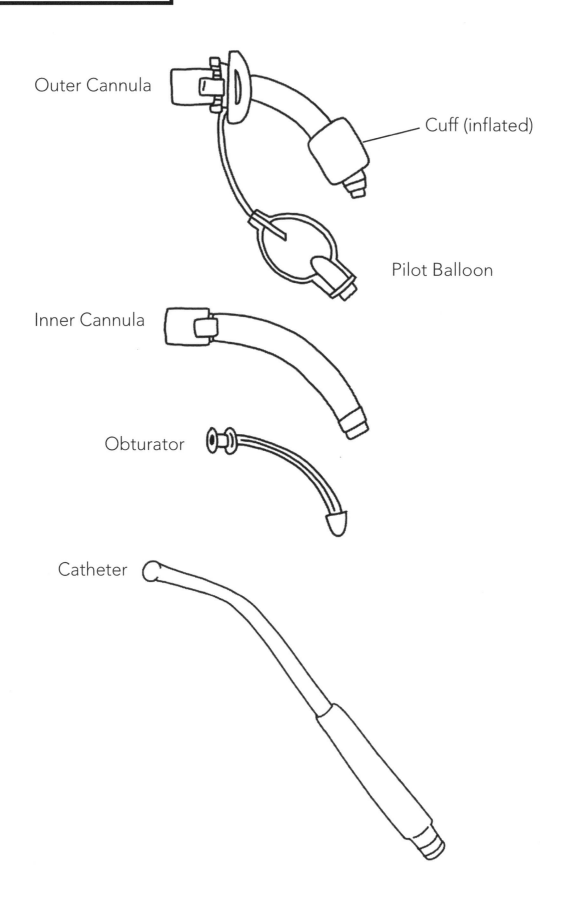

Speaking Valve

The PassyMuir® Valve (PMV) is a popular speaking valve (Passy Muir, Inc., n.d.) *PMVs are usually purple, although they also come in white, clear, and aqua blue. PMVs are easy to place and remove. Review the PMV website for thorough instructions* (Pleton, 2015).

SAFETY.
- Always deflate the trach cuff before placing a valve. Never use with a foam-filled, cuffed trach tube.
- Monitor the patient's vitals throughout. Remove the valve immediately if the patient has difficulty breathing.
- Clean using warm, soapy water. Rinse thoroughly with warm water. Don't use peroxide, bleach, vinegar, alcohol, brushes, or cotton swabs to clean the PMV. Air dry only.

PLACING A PMV.
1. Position the patient in a comfortable, upright posture.
   - Never use while sleeping (John Hopkins, n.d.-b).
2. Wash your hands with antibacterial soap and dry with a clean paper towel or electric dryer. Put on clean gloves.
3. Suction the trach (and the mouth and nose as needed) while monitoring the patient's vitals. Provide breaks and oxygen as needed.
4. Deflate the cuff (if the patient has one, see page 20).
   - Continue to monitor vitals.
5. Suction more if needed.
6. Hold the neck plate (flange) in place with one hand.

DYSPHAGIA

Page 2 of 2

7. Place the speaking valve at the end of the trach tube and twist it clockwise (to the right) for one-quarter turn.

It is common for patients to cough after the speaking valve is placed. Occasionally, they may cough hard enough for the speaking valve to pop off. In that case, suction the trach as needed, clean the speaking valve as needed, and place the speaking valve on again.

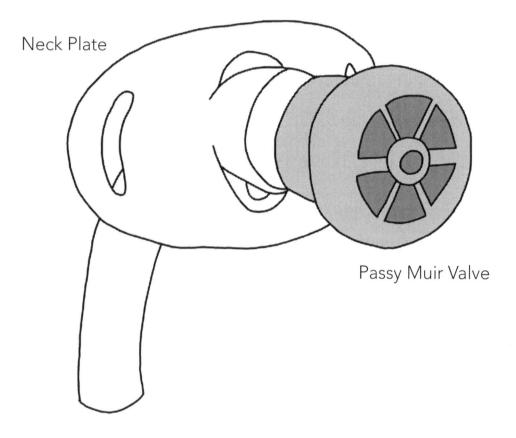

DYSPHAGIA

Modified Barium Swallowing Study

A modified barium swallowing study (MBSS) is an outpatient X-ray examination that helps determine how well you chew and swallow. It takes about 10 minutes to complete. It is one of the best ways to see if and why you are aspirating on food or liquids.

- MBSS usually takes place in a hospital's radiology suite. A speech therapist, radiologist or technician, and maybe a nurse will be present. You will be asked to sit down next to the X-ray machine. The radiologist will be standing to your side, controlling the X-ray. The speech therapist will stand nearby and hand you different food and drinks to consume.

- The therapist will ask you to eat foods of various textures, all of which will be coated in barium. Barium is a substance that can be seen on X-rays, making it possible for the team to see exactly where the food travels in your mouth and throat. It is safe to consume and does not have a distinctive flavor, though some people describe it as "chalky." Your therapist will also ask you to drink liquid barium.

DYSPHAGIA

- You will get the results of the study right away. The therapist may give you suggestions for how to improve your chewing and swallowing. They may tell you which food and drinks are safe to eat and which to avoid. They may also give you safe swallowing strategies and exercises to strengthen your face and throat muscles.

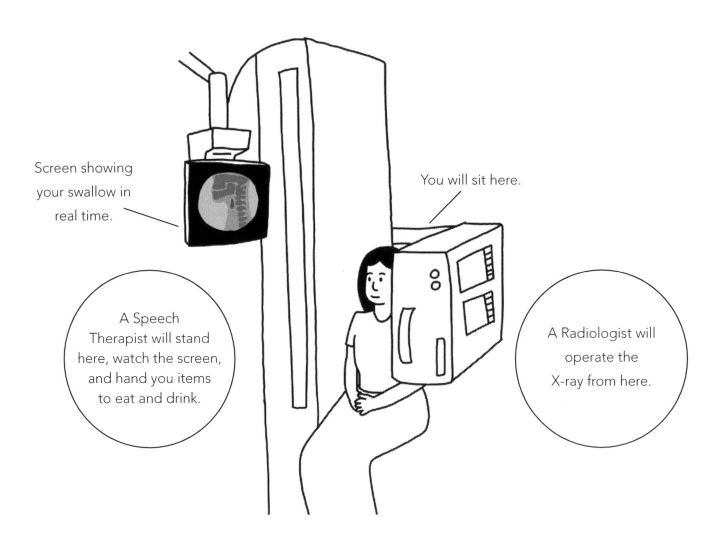

DYSPHAGIA

FEES

A fiberoptic endoscopic evaluation of swallowing (FEES) is an outpatient examination. It examines the structure and function of your throat and how safely you swallow. It takes about 20 minutes to complete.

- The speech therapist or otolaryngologist (ENT doctor) will insert a flexible endoscope, about the width of a spaghetti noddle, in your nostril and then partway down your throat. On the tip of the endoscope is a camera and a light.

- The therapist will be controlling the tip of the endoscope, and you may feel it slightly as it moves in your throat. You may feel the urge to swallow more than usual.

- You will then be asked to eat and drink. The therapist will look for left-over food or liquid in your throat or for food or liquid spilling into your airway (aspiration).

- You will get the results of the study right away. The therapist may give you suggestions for how to improve your chewing and swallowing. They may tell you which foods are safe to eat and which foods to avoid. They may also give you safe swallowing strategies and exercises to strengthen your face and throat muscles.

DYSPHAGIA

Page 2 of 2

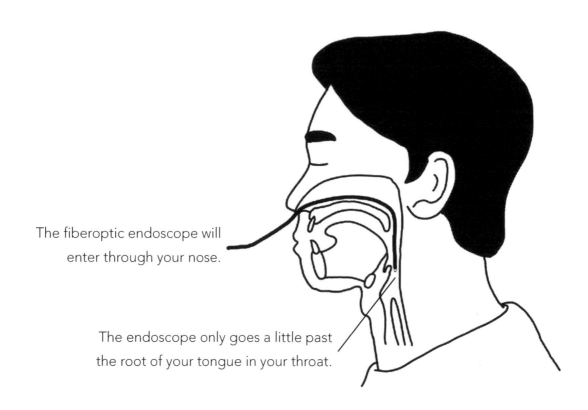

DYSPHAGIA

Oral Hygiene

Good oral hygiene prevents more than tooth decay and gingivitis. It also helps prevent thrush (a fungal infection in the mouth) and aspiration pneumonia (an infection in the lungs caused by inhaling food or drinks).

- Use a toothbrush with soft bristles and toothpaste.
- Brush your teeth and tongue once in the morning and once in the evening.
- Floss before you go to bed.
- Use alcohol-free and sugar-free mouthwash, if you choose to use mouthwash.
- Visit the dentist every 6 months.
- Treat xerostomia (dry mouth) by sipping on water throughout the day.
    - 1/3 of all adults over the age of 65 experience dry mouth *(American Dental Association, 2019)*.
- Avoid alcohol, caffeine, and sugary drinks.

DYSPHAGIA

Anatomy & Physiology

Chewing and swallowing use dozens of muscles. All of these muscles must coordinate precisely in order for you to eat and drink.

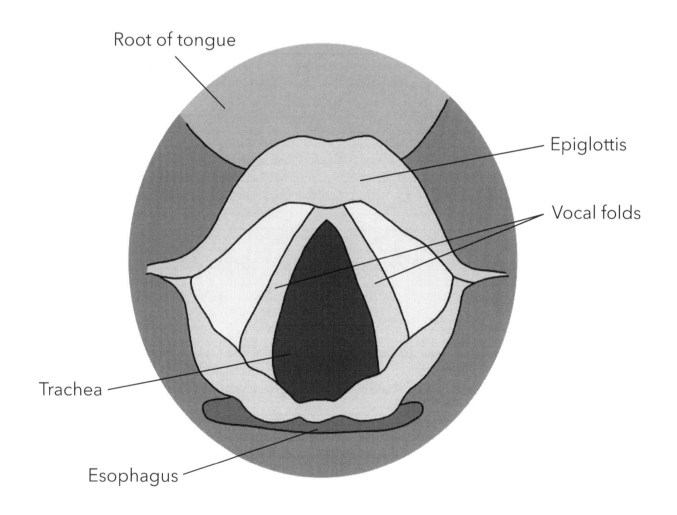

Eagle-eye view of the vocal folds and trachea.

DYSPHAGIA

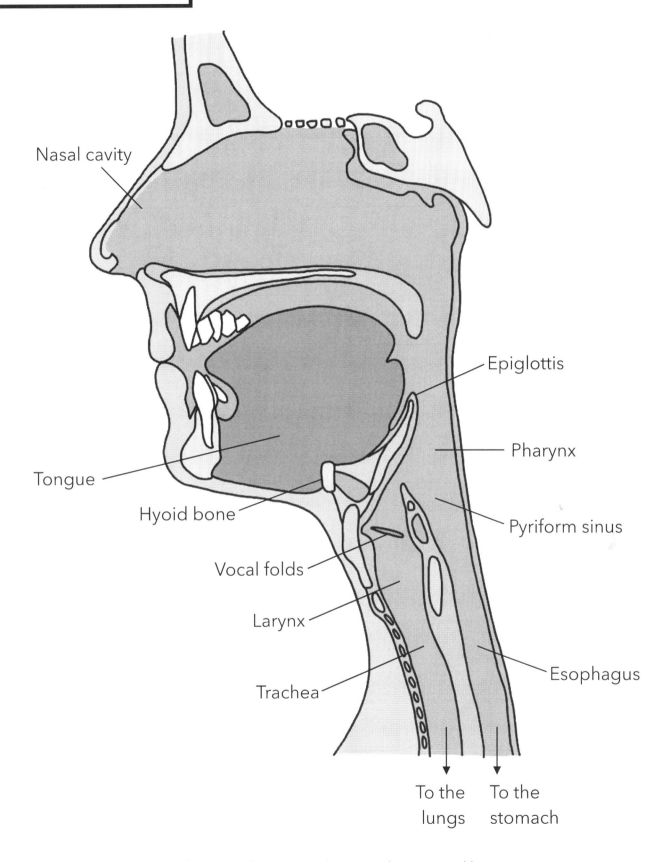

Side-view of the nasal cavity, oral cavity, pharynx, and larynx.

DYSPHAGIA

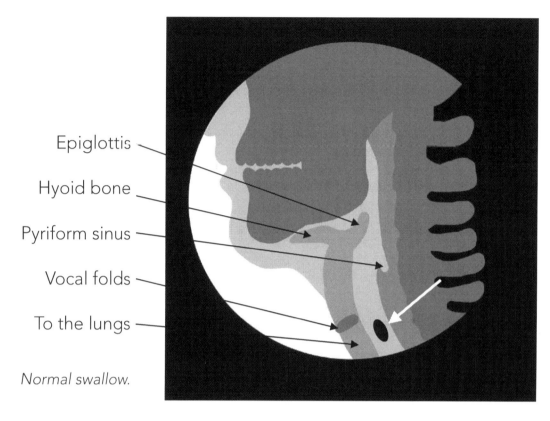

Normal swallow.

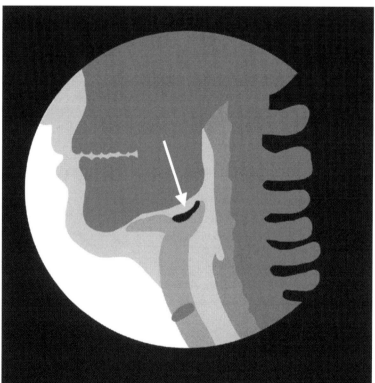

Residue in the valleculae.

DYSPHAGIA

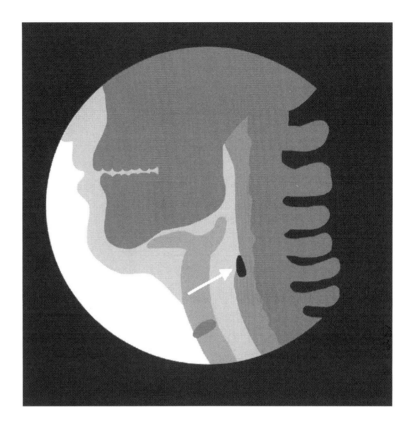

Residue in the pyriform sinus.

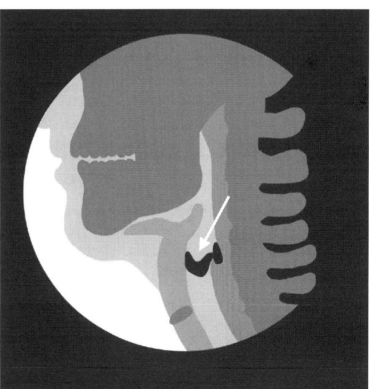

Residue in the pyriform sinus with spillage.

DYSPHAGIA

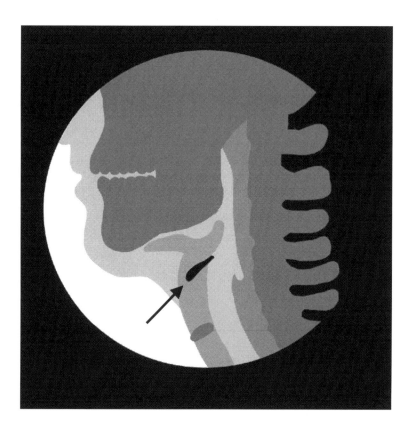

Laryngeal penetration.

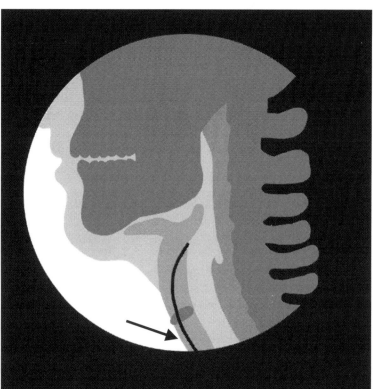

Aspiration.

DYSPHAGIA

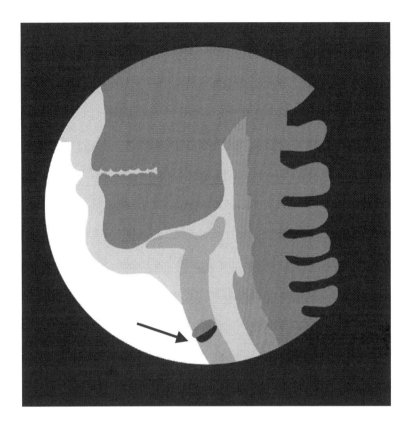

Residue beneath the vocal folds.

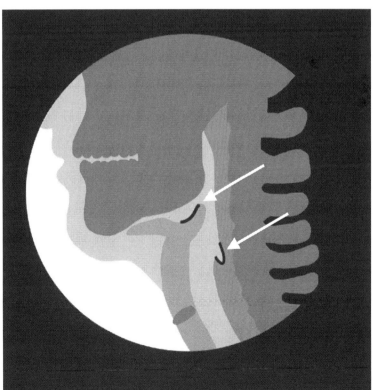

Residue in the valleculae and pyriform sinus.

MEMORY

Memory is the encoding, storing, and recall of information. It includes working, short term, long term, and everyday recall. The goal of treatment is to increase memory skills and/or develop compensations in order to increase quality of life and independence. Choose memory goals and techniques based on the patient's previous and current levels of functioning, nature of the memory disorder (i.e., acute or progressive), amount of support available, motivation, insight into deficits, and other relevant factors.

Memory treatment includes:
- Restorative treatment (e.g. increased ability to remember people's names)
- Compensatory treatment (e.g. writing down appointment reminders)

MEMORY

Therapist Instructions

EVALUATIONS. Consider using memory screens, parts of formal cognitive evaluations, and/or informal cognitive-linguistic evaluations versus a full cognitive battery. Cognitive batteries can take hours to complete which is precious time for those patients with limited health insurance coverage.

- Memory screens include the *Montreal Cognitive Assessment* (MoCA), *Short Blessed Test*, *Mini-Mental State Evaluation* (MMSE), *Saint Louis University Mental Status* (SLUMS), *Addenbrooke's Cognitive Examination*, and *Mini-Cog*.
- Formal batteries include the *Ross Information Processing Assessment*. There is also a geriatric version for patients aged 55 years and up.
- Informal cognitive-linguistic evaluations often include questions about basic orientation, long term memory, short term memory, and recalling information from reading material.

DAY ONE OF TREATMENT. Provide the following handouts, as needed.

- Homework Log, Memory Impairments, Forgetfulness, How to Avoid Memory Loss, Memory Strategies, Ways to Improve Memory, Spaced Retrieval, Memory Books, Daily Journal, Monthly Calendar, Therapy Team, Brain Organization Tips, Remembering Appointments.
- Highlight key points on the handouts, then review with your patients. Ask questions to make sure they understand the content. Answer any questions they may have.

MEMORY STRATEGIES (PAGE 92) VS. WAYS TO IMPROVE MEMORY (PAGE 93). The Memory Strategies handout is a compact version of the Ways to Improve Memory handout. The Memory Strategies can be a good starting point for patients with more severe memory impairments.

- Review the strategies from either handout with your patients and ask, "Which strategies do you already use? Which are you interested in trying?" Practice the strategies while completing the memory tasks in this chapter.

MEMORY

USING THE WAYS TO IMPROVE MEMORY (PAGE 95). For patients with milder memory deficits who would benefit from completing practical tasks.

SPACED RETRIEVAL (PAGE 99). Trial this technique with your patient first. If it seems to help them remember new information, provide caregiver training.

MEMORY BOOKS (PAGE 101) & WALLETS (PAGE 110). Provide the caregiver with the Memory Book Contents handout and a copy of the template (make extra copies of page 106 as needed). Review instructions.
- Patients who carry their purse or wallet with them everywhere may benefit from the memory wallet instead.
- Follow up with the caregiver every few days to check on the progress of the memory book/wallet.

MEDICATIONS. Obtain the latest copy of the patient's medication list. Ask the patient to fill out the My Medications form (page 116).
- Many medications have both a generic name and a brand name. Ask the patient to write down the name most familiar to them.
- Turn this into an ongoing memory task by asking your patient questions such as, "What is xxx medication used for?" or "What is the name of your blood pressure pill?" etc.

DAILY JOURNAL (PAGE 117). To cue for a more detailed journal entry, say "Tell me everything you did today" or "What's the very first thing you did today? And then what happened?" etc.

SCHEDULES (PAGES 118–119). Use with patients who struggle to keep track of their daily schedule, would benefit from getting on a routine, or would like to keep track of personal goals. Breaking down their day into larger chunks (included in these worksheets) can help.

MEMORY

THE CALENDAR TASKS (PAGE 122–131). For ease of use, copy the Calendar Tasks one-sided.
- Ask the patient to review the calendar for about a minute before answering the questions. If they can't remember a detail, then encourage them to check the calendar and avoid guessing.
- Encourage them to add only pertinent information and to cross out each instruction right after adding it to the calendar.
- Generalize this task by asking them to write down all of their therapy appointments on a calendar. Monitor their adherence and follow up as needed.
- Increase the difficulty of these tasks by asking the patient to review and memorize what they just wrote down using their memory strategies.

THERAPY TEAM (PAGE 136). Either you or your patient can fill out this form. Turn it into a memory task by using the tips from the Remembering People's Names handout.

NAMES TO PICTURES/PHOTOS TASKS (PAGES 137–142). Use with the Remembering People's Names handout as needed (page 134). The same set of people are used twice: Once with the name written directly under the picture, and once without the name. First ask your patient to memorize the people's names with the written cues. To increase the challenge, next present the page without the names.

BRAIN ORGANIZATION TIPS (PAGE 155). Practice these tips with your patient during practical tasks.

REMEMBERING INSTRUCTIONS (PAGE 156). Expand the challenge by prompting the patient to take notes while you read aloud. See the Aphasia and Visual Neglect chapters for additional reading material.

APPOINTMENT NOTES (PAGE 160). Use the Appointment Notes worksheet for medical appointments or even therapy sessions.

MEMORY

ATTENTION TREATMENT. Attention can be difficult to isolate and measure because several cognitive processes may impact each task.
- To measure attention:
    - Count how many cues the patient needed to remain on task during a specific time period.
    - Measure the type (e.g., verbal, written, etc.) and frequency (e.g., rare, intermittent, frequent, etc.) of cues for attention the patient needed to complete a variety of tasks, such as reading comprehension, auditory comprehension, and completing mental math.
- While treatment planning, figure out which cognitive processes (e.g., attention or memory) are required to complete each task, then decide what process you will record.
    - Be consistent with which cognitive process you decide to focus on.
    - If you measure attention via the number of cues needed during a mental math task, then continue to measure attention every time the patient completes a mental math task. Don't record the number of cues needed as a measure of memory one week and then attention the next week.

THINGS TO REMEMBER.
- Dates are abbreviated in the American format of MM/DD/YY.
- Some tasks include two pages. Print these one-sided (so the patient doesn't need to flip the paper back and forth).
- Patients may not realize that they have a memory impairment until after you've completed your evaluation with them. They may be shocked, sad, and even berate themselves. Take this opportunity to educate them. The brain can heal, and neuroplasticity is on their side (see page 24).
- Frequently refer back to the patient's calendar and strategies during your time together in speech therapy.
- Whenever you can, incorporate materials from the patient's life. For example, ask a patient to read a menu, memorize their order, and then place it using the facility's phone. Or use the novel the patient is already reading to read aloud and summarize.

MEMORY

Contents

Memory Impairments............................	88
Forgetfulness......................................	90
How to Avoid Memory Loss...................	91
Memory Strategies..............................	92
Ways to Improve Memory.....................	93
Using the Ways to Improve Memory..........	95
Orientation..	98
Spaced Retrieval................................	99
Memory Books...................................	101
Memory Book Example Pages.........	102
Memory Book Contents.................	103
Template..................................	104
Memory Wallet Overview.......................	110
Template..................................	111
Remembering Your Medications..............	114
Medication List Instructions...................	115
My Medications...................................	116
Daily Journal......................................	117
Create a Schedule...............................	118
Daily Schedule...................................	119
Monthly Calendar *(Overview)*.................	120
Monthly Calendar.......................	121
Reading a Calendar.............................	122
Write In Appointments.........................	126
Make Associations..............................	132
Remembering People's Names...............	134
Therapy Team....................................	136

MEMORY

Names to Pictures..................................	137
Names to Photos..................................	141
Passwords...	143
Group & Memorize................................	144
Memorize Lists.....................................	146
Memorize Lists *(Task)*...........................	148
Brain Organization Tips........................	155
Remembering Instructions....................	156
Remembering Appointments.................	158
Neurology Appointments......................	159
Appointment Notes.....................	160
Memos & Appointments.......................	161
Remembering Reading Material.............	165

SEE ALSO

Neuroplasticity...........................	24
Neuroanatomy & Physiology..........	189
Paragraphs................................	389
Reading.....................................	395

MEMORY

Memory Impairments

The types of memory impairments include:

MILD COGNITIVE IMPAIRMENT. Difficulties with memory, language, and thinking abilities that are more severe than can be explained by normal aging but less severe than dementia.

DEMENTIA. Dementia is an umbrella term for a group of symptoms. It is memory loss **plus** difficulties in one (or more) of the following: judgment, abstract reasoning, visuospatial, executive functioning, and/or language.
- **Alzheimer's Disease**: The most common form of dementia. It is caused by beta-amyloid plaque buildup and tau protein tangles that lead to brain cell death. This usually starts in the hippocampus, the memory center of the brain.
- **Lewy Body Dementia**: The second most common form of dementia. It is caused by abnormal plaque buildup in the brain, called Lewy bodies.

CEREBROVASCULAR ACCIDENT (CVA, Stroke). Caused by a blockage of blood flow to the brain or a ruptured blood vessel in the brain. Both lead to brain cell death. Intensive therapy can help create new brain cell pathways. This improves function, especially in the first 6 months after the stroke *(Pruski, 2021)*.

MEMORY

TRAUMATIC BRAIN INJURY. Caused by a sudden and violent blow to the brain, such as a fall, car accident, gunshot wound, or blunt force trauma.

ENCEPHALOPATHY. An umbrella term for any dysfunction of the brain. It may cause memory impairments.

BRAIN TUMORS. Tumors can cause neurological changes, including memory impairments. The changes depend on the location and size of the tumors.

MEMORY

Forgetfulness

Some forgetfulness is normal. Normal forgetfulness can be caused by aging, stress, depression, diabetes, thyroid disease, Vitamin B-12 deficiency, and medication side effects (Berkley, 2006). But other types of memory loss are abnormal. Contact your doctor if you notice signs of abnormal memory loss.

NORMAL FORGETFULNESS. These signs happen once in a while.
- The "tip of the tongue" feeling while talking
- Forgetting some details of an event
- Forgetting the name of the person you just met
- Forgetting your passwords
- Forgetting why you went into another room
- Forgetting where you parked your car
- Forgetting appointments

ABNORMAL MEMORY LOSS. These signs happen often and become more severe over time.
- Feeling confused doing familiar tasks
- Forgetting entire events that just happened
- Forgetting how to use common objects, like a calculator or calendar
- Forgetting the current month or year
- Close family members and friends become worried about your memory

> MEMORY

How to Avoid Memory Loss

Neuropsychologists and neurologists recommend using the following tips to avoid memory loss.

EAT RIGHT.
- Eat a balanced diet *(Mayo Clinic Staff, 2021)*.
- Limit fried foods, desserts, and frozen dinners.

EXERCISE.
- Complete your therapy exercises.
- Take walks or go to the gym at least 30 minutes per day, 3 days a week.

MENTAL EXERCISE.
- Do brain games.
- Read, play cards, play word games, and do puzzles.

SOCIALIZE.
- Meet new people, attend events, host dinners, write emails and letters to family and friends, join a club, visit the Senior Center.

MEMORY

Memory Strategies

Use these tips to help you remember new information.

WRITE IT DOWN.
- Take notes. Use a calendar to help you remember appointments.

REPEAT, REPEAT, REPEAT.
- Say what you want to remember, such as a person's name, over and over again.

TAKE MENTAL PICTURES.
- Visualize what you want to remember, such as where you left your keys.
- Take a mental snapshot and store it away in your brain *(Axelrod, 2016)*.

USE ASSOCIATIONS.
- Connect what you want to remember with what you already know *(Kelly & O'Sullivan, 2015)*.

USE GROUPS.
- Organize what you want to remember into smaller groups, such as your grocery list by produce and canned foods.

Ways to Improve Memory

PAY ATTENTION. Listen, look, and focus on what you want to remember *(Cleveland Clinic, 2019)*.

USE MENTAL PICTURES. Take a mental picture and store it in your brain. For example, visualize where you left your keys and take a mental picture.

REPEAT AND REHEARSE. Repeat over and over what you have just learned, such as a new name or phone number.

CHUNK AND ORGANIZE INFO. Sort information into categories. For example, organize your grocery list into groups, such as produce and canned foods.

CREATE ASSOCIATIONS. Make connections between what you want to remember and what you already know. For example, remember a new name by connecting it to someone with the same name.

MEMORY

USE EXTERNAL AIDS. Wear a watch, use a planner or calendar to help you keep a schedule, or write a checklist to remember grocery items.

ADAPT YOUR ENVIRONMENT. Remove background noise and clutter.

KEEP ITEMS IN THE SAME PLACE. Have containers or places where items 'belong', such as a key rack by the door or a file box for important papers.

HAVE A ROUTINE. Have a set schedule for waking up, meals, naps, bedtime, etc. to get your body into a routine. This helps with memory *(Heerema, 2020)*.

IMPROVE YOUR OVERALL HEALTH. Go for a walk, eat healthy fruits and vegetables, and drink plenty of water. This improves brain function and brain cell production *(Harvard Health Publishing, 2016)*.

SOCIALIZE AND CONTINUE YOUR HOBBIES. Host dinners, call old friends, join a club. Keep up with hobbies such as reading, gardening, and listening to music.

DO ACTIVITIES THAT IMPROVE MEMORY. Play board games, card games, crossword puzzles, word searches, and sudoku puzzles. Read the newspaper, write e-mails, work on the computer, etc.

Using the Ways to Improve Memory

Below are practical ways to use your memory strategies.

WRITE IT DOWN.
- Take notes during appointments.
- Keep a daily journal.
- Use a calendar or planner to write down appointments.
- Jot down people's names.
- Make a copy of your medication list.
- Make to-do lists, grocery lists, exercise lists, etc.
- Use your phone for appointments, reminders, timers, and alarms.
- Use *Amazon Echo™* for appointments, reminders, timers, and alarms.
- Use these worksheets: Daily Journal, Create a Schedule, Monthly Calendar, Remembering People's Names, Memorize Lists, Remembering Appointments, Memos & Appointments.

REPEAT, REPEAT, REPEAT.
- Immediately after meeting a person, say their name twice.
- Repeat information back to the person who gave it to you. Then repeat it to yourself.
    - *For example, "Do my exercises twice a day, do my exercises twice a day."*

MEMORY

- Memorize lists by repeating them over and over.
- Remember reading material by summarizing what you read immediately after you read it.
- Learn how to use a new piece of technology by repeating the same action over and over again.
    - *For example, set up and delete a new alarm on your phone. Repeat the steps at least 3 times in a row.*
- Use these worksheets: Medication List, Remembering People's Names, Names to Pictures, Memorize Lists, Remembering Instructions, Memos & Appointments.

TAKE MENTAL PICTURES.

- To remember where you put an item, place the item where it belongs and then take note of what's around it.
    - *For example, "I placed the keys in the brown dish. The yellow flowers are to the right and the white wall is behind it."*
- To remember written information, take note of where the information is located on the paper.
    - *For example, "The paragraph I want to remember is on the bottom of the first page of the colorful brochure."*
- To remember where you parked your car, take note of its location in relation to the store you're visiting.
    - *For example, "My car is parked in the middle of the parking lot. The lane is lined up with the logo of the store."*
- Use these worksheets: Make Associations, Names to Photos, Group & Memorize.

MEMORY

USE ASSOCIATIONS.

- Remember someone's name by connecting it to someone else with the same or similar name.
- Memorize the purpose of your prescription medication by creating a simple or funny phrase.
    - *For example, "Am**LO**dipine **LOW**ers blood pressure"*
    - *Or, "Simva**STAT**in helps with **FAT** 'n cholesterol"*
    - *Or, "**HYDRO**chlorothiazide is my **WATER** pill"*
- Use these worksheets: Medication List, Make Associations, Remembering People's Names, Names to Pictures.

USE GROUPS.

- Organize your grocery list by group or by their location in the store.
    - *For example, "I need 3 items from dairy, 2 from meat, and 5 from the canned food aisle."*
- Memorize your entire list of medications by grouping them. Group by when you take them or what they're used for.
- Recall what you just read by stopping regularly and summarizing the information.
- Use these worksheets: Medication List, Group & Memorize, Memorize Lists.

MEMORY

Orientation

Use this worksheet everyday with patients who have acute brain injuries. Ask all of the questions first, then provide orientation treatment as needed.

1. What is your name? _____
2. What is your birthdate? _____
3. Where do you live? _____
4. What time is it? _____
5. What day of the week is it? _____
6. What month is it? _____
7. What is today's date? _____
8. What year is it? _____
9. Why were you at the hospital? _____
   _____
10. What symptoms are you experiencing? _____
    _____

Today's date _____   Today's Score (correct) _____/10

MEMORY

Spaced Retrieval

Use this technique to help your loved one remember new information (Landauer & Bjork, 1978).

They can use Spaced Retrieval to remember appointments, for orientation information ("Where are we now?"), and to answer repetitive questions ("When will we go home?")

ASK THE QUESTION. Ask your loved one a specific, open-ended question (cannot be answered by "yes" or "no").
- *For example, "When is your eye appointment?"*
- *Or, "Where do you live?"*
- *Or, "Why were you in the hospital?"*

GIVE THE CORRECT RESPONSE.
- *For example, "Tuesday at 10 am."*
- *Or, "June Fields Retirement Home."*
- *Or, "I broke my hip."*

ASK THE QUESTION AGAIN. Ask the exact same question again and wait for a response. The answer should exactly mimic your correct response ("Tuesday at 10 am").
- If your loved one was **incorrect**, then go back to the first step.
- If your loved one was **correct**, then wait 15 seconds and ask the exact same question again.

MEMORY

WAIT, THEN ASK AGAIN. Continue to increase the time between asking the question again. Start with 15 seconds, then increase the time to 30 seconds, 60 seconds, 2 minutes, 4 minutes, 8 minutes, etc. You may go up to half an hour or beyond.
- Remember, the response must be correct to increase the time interval. If incorrect, go back to the first step.

If your loved one has a hard time with a question, try rewording it. Or try a different response. User fewer and simpler words.

MEMORY

Memory Books

HOW TO USE A MEMORY BOOK
- Memory books are meant to be a fun sharing experience. They can increase mood and quality of life (Elfrink et al., 2018).
- Slowly flip through the book. Encourage conversation by pointing to photos and asking open-ended questions
  - "Who is this? Where was this photo taken?"
- Give reminders to read captions. This helps your loved one remember information.
- Avoid "quizzing" your loved one. Instead, give opportunities to share parts of their life story.
- Memory books can also be used to answer any repetitive questions your loved one may ask. For example, if they frequently ask, "When are we going home?" prompt them to open the memory book and find the answer under Location Information.

HOW TO FORMAT A MEMORY BOOK
- Include photos whenever possible. Add short captions as needed.
- Place photos and text on plain white printer paper.
- Include headings and page numbers on each page.
- Write or type using large text (24 points or larger).
- Limit text to 3-4 short sentences on each page. Use bullet points.
- Laminate or place paper in plastic protective sleeves. Keep the book in a 3-ring binder or photo album.

MEMORY

Memory Book Example Pages

Dooneese Marelly

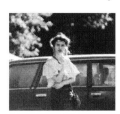

Me in the 1960's.

1. I was born in Buffalo, New York.
2. My birthday is June 1, 1945.
3. I grew up on my grandparent's farm in the Finger Lakes.

PAGE 2

Dooneese's Family

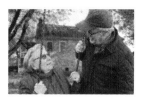

Mom and Papa at their cabin in Michigan.

1. My parents were Mary and John.
2. Mom was a bank teller and singer.
3. Papa was a farmer.

PAGE 3

Dooneese's Home

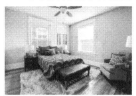

This is my room.
My room number is 123.

1. I live in Arizona.
2. I live in a retirement home called "June Meadows."
3. I moved here in 2019.

PAGE 12

Dooneese's Schedule

8:30 AM: Wake Up

9:30 AM: Breakfast

10:15 AM: Arts & Crafts

11:30 AM: Lunch

12:30 PM: Outing

4:00 PM: TV or Games

5:30 PM: Dinner

6:30 PM: Shower

9:00 PM: Bedtime

PAGE 13

MEMORY

Memory Book Contents

COVER. See template on page 104.

TABLE OF CONTENTS. Page 105.

BASIC PAGE. Page 106, can include the following:
- Personal information: full name, date of birth, birth place, fond childhood memories, career, hobbies and talents, memorable happy events (vacations, buying a new car, winning an award, etc.)
- Careers, hobbies, traits, the names of children, parents, pets, and friends, etc.
- Location: current residence ("retirement home" or "Bobby's house") and previous residences
- Medical history: diagnoses, recent hospitalizations, and/or surgeries

SCHEDULE. Page 107, include wake up time, breakfast, reading hour, etc.

EMERGENCY MEDICAL INFORMATION. Page 108.

MEDICATION LIST. Page 109.

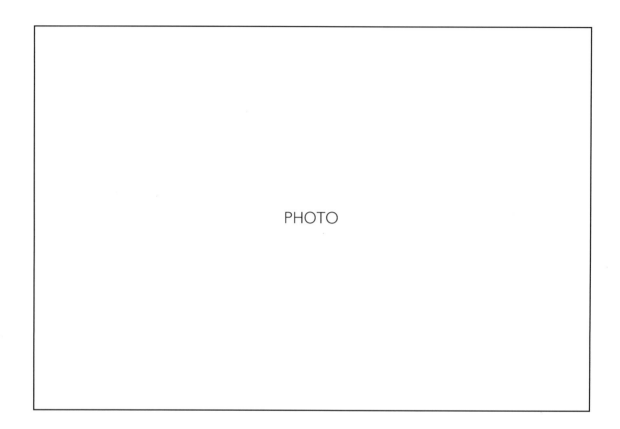

NAME OF PATIENT

Memory Book

Table of Contents

_____ Page _____

_____ _____

_____ _____

_____ _____

_____ _____

_____ _____

_____ _____

_____ _____

_____ _____

_____ _____

_____ _____

_____ _____

TITLE OF PAGE

[PHOTO]

PHOTO CAPTION

_____
_____
_____
_____
_____

1-3 SHORT AND SIMPLE SENTENCES

Page _____

_____ Schedule
NAME OF PATIENT

TIME	EVENT
_____	_____
_____	_____
_____	_____
_____	_____
_____	_____
_____	_____
_____	_____
_____	_____

Page _____

Emergency Medical Information

Name: _____

Birthdate: _____/_____/_____ Age: _____

Allergies: _____

Primary Care Physician: _____

    Phone number: _____

Emergency Contact: _____

    Phone number: _____

Emergency Contact: _____

    Phone number: _____

Medical Conditions: _____

_____

Surgical History: _____

Page ____

Medications

Updated: _____ / _____ / _____

Medication	Dosage

Page ___

MEMORY

Memory Wallets

Memory wallets are just like memory books, only smaller. Wallet-sized, to be precise! They're meant to be easy to carry around in place of a memory book if your loved one prefers to keep a memory aid in their wallet.

- Training for a memory wallet will be the same as a memory book.
- Extra training includes spaced retrieval and other strategies to remember to always keep it in a pocket or purse.
- Memory wallet pages should have less text than a memory book. This makes the smaller format easier to read.
- Use a font size (14 points or larger) that your loved one can easily read.

See the following pages for templates. Copy then cut out along the dotted line:
- Page 111: Fill in the Blank
- Page 112: Empty Template
- Page 113: Photos and Captions

My name is My birthday is I was born in	I live at I have lived here for
My spouse is	My children are
My hobbies are	My favorite things are
My fondest memory is	My favorite holiday is
My medications are	My medical history is

| (front) PHOTO WITH CAPTION BELOW | (back) PHOTO WITH CAPTION BELOW |

| (front) PHOTO WITH CAPTION TO THE RIGHT | | (back) PHOTO WITH CAPTION TO THE RIGHT | |

(front) PHOTO WITH CAPTION ON THE BACK

(front) PHOTO WITH CAPTION ON THE BACK

The Adult Speech Therapy Workbook © 2021 Chung Hwa Brewer

> MEMORY

Remembering Your Medications

KEEP A ROUTINE. Take your medications at the same time and place every day.

MAKE A LIST of all of your medications. Include what they're for, the dosage, and what time of day you should take each. See page 116 for a template.

USE A PILL BOX. Have all your medications ready.

PLACE REMINDER NOTES where you'll see them (e.g., on the bathroom door, refrigerator door, coffee pot, etc.)

USE ALARMS. Program your phone or *Alexa™* device to sound an alarm whenever it's time to take your medications.

USE A CALENDAR. Write reminders to take your medications. Cross them out only **after** you've taken them. Add to your calendar when to call for a prescription refill (at least one week before running out).

MEMORY

Medication List Instructions

Use the following template to organize your medications in one place. List the medications chronologically, with your morning medications listed first and your evening medications after. Add your "as needed" or "PRN" medications to the end of the list.

NAME. Generic or brand name, whichever one is easier for you to remember.

DOSAGE. Number of pills, mg, or units.

PURPOSE: Reason for taking the medication.
- *For example, "blood pressure," "anti-seizure," or "diabetes."*

TIMES TAKEN. AM, Noon, PM, as needed, after breakfast, with meals, before bed, Monday/Wednesday/Friday, etc.

My Medications

Date Updated: _____

Name	Dosage	Purpose	Times Taken *List chronologically*

MEMORY

Daily Journal

At the end of each day, fill out this form with as much detail as possible.

Today's date is _____

What I did today

_____

_____

_____

Who I saw today

_____

_____

_____

How I felt today

_____

_____

_____

MEMORY

Create a Schedule

Write in the times that you typically do the following activities. Fill in the rest of your schedule. For example, "10 AM, Volunteering" or "4 PM, Pick up the kids."

_____   Wake up
_____

_____   Breakfast
_____

_____   _____

_____   _____

_____   _____

_____   Lunch
_____

_____   _____

_____   _____

_____   Go to bed
_____

Daily Schedule

Having a routine improves memory and keeps your organized.

Time   **Activity**

_____   _____

_____   _____

_____   _____

_____   _____

_____   _____

_____   _____

_____   _____

_____   _____

_____   _____

_____   _____

MEMORY

Monthly Calendar

Use this calendar to stay organized and keep track of important events.

TIPS FOR USING THE CALENDAR.
- Fill out the dates for the entire month.
- Add birthdays, anniversaries, and holidays.
- Add appointments and bill due dates.
- Add any other important events.
- Cross out the days as each day passes.

FOLLOW-UP QUESTIONS USING THE CALENDAR.
1. What year is it?
2. What month is it?
3. What day of the week is it?
4. What is today's date?
5. What holidays are celebrated this month?
6. What day of the week is the first?
7. What day of the week does the month end on?
8. What birthdays are in this month?
9. How many Sundays are in this month?
10. What is the date one week from today?

MONTH: _____ **YEAR:** _____

Sunday	Monday	Tuesday	Wednesday	Thursday	Friday	Saturday

MEMORY

Page 1 of 2

Reading a Calendar

Use the calendar on the next page to answer the questions.

---

1. What day of the week is May 10th? _____

2. What date is the first Saturday? _____

3. What day of the week is the last day of the month? _____

4. When is the dentist appointment? _____

5. Is the X-ray before or after the dentist appointment? _____

6. When is mom's birthday? _____

7. How long after her birthday is her party? _____

8. What day of the week does June start on? _____

9. What time is the X-ray appointment? _____

10. What day of the week is the first? _____

MEMORY

Page 2 of 2

May

Sunday	Monday	Tuesday	Wednesday	Thursday	Friday	Saturday
1	2	3	4	5	6	7
8	9 Dentist 7:45 am	10	11	12 X-Ray 11:00 am	13	14
15	16	17	18	19	20 Mom's Birthday	21 Mom's Party 6:00 pm
22	23	24	25	26	27	28
29	30	31				

MEMORY

Reading a Calendar

Use the calendar on the next page to answer the questions.

---

1. What day of the week is the first? _____

2. When is the BBQ? _____

3. Is the bank visit scheduled before the departure? _____

4. How many days long is the trip? _____

5. What event happens during the trip? _____

6. What day of the week is the bank visit? _____

7. How many Saturdays are there this month? _____

8. How many Sundays are there this month? _____

9. What day of the week does June end on? _____

10. What day of the week does August start on? _____

MEMORY

July

Sunday	Monday	Tuesday	Wednesday	Thursday	Friday	Saturday
					1	2
3	4 BBQ 3 pm	5	6	7	8	9
10	11	12	13	14 Bank 9:00 am	15 Depart 6:30 am	16
17 50th Anniversary!	18	19 Return 7:00 pm	20	21	22	23
24/31	25	26	27	28	29	30

MEMORY

Write In Appointments

Add the following events to the calendar on the next page.

---

1. You return from Hawaii on the 2nd at 8:30 pm.
2. Your cousin is visiting from the 5th to the 7th.
3. David's birthday is on the 31st.
4. Your dentist appointment is at 10:15 am on the 17th.
5. Your meeting at the bank is at 10:00 am on the 22nd.

MEMORY

Page 2 of 2

			January			
Sunday	Monday	Tuesday	Wednesday	Thursday	Friday	Saturday
	1	2	3	4	5	6
7	8	9	10	11	12	13
14	15	16	17	18	19	20
21	22	23	24	25	26	27
28	29	30	31			

MEMORY

Write In Appointments

Add the following events to the calendar on the next page.

---

1. Easter Sunday is on the 18th.//
2. The Easter Party is on Friday the 16th at 7 pm.
3. Yolanda's baby, Jose, is turning 1 on the 1st.
4. Jose's birthday party is on the 3rd at 1:00 pm.
5. The package from England should be arriving on the 24th.

MEMORY

Page 2 of 2

			April			
Sunday	Monday	Tuesday	Wednesday	Thursday	Friday	Saturday
				1	2	3
4	5	6	7	8	9	10
11	12	13	14	15	16	17
18	19	20	21	22	23	24
25	26	27	28	29	30	

MEMORY

Write In Appointments

Add the following events to the calendar on the next page.

---

1. You have a post-op follow-up appointment with Dr. Downey on Friday the 10th at 9:30 am.

2. Martha is coming to visit from Florida on the last Tuesday of the month.

3. Your surgery is scheduled for the 3rd at 7:30 am. Don't eat or drink after midnight the previous day.

4. The kids are visiting on the weekend after your surgery.

5. Date with Laura on February 14 at D'Angelo's Bistro in Downtown.

MEMORY

Page 2 of 2

			February			
Sunday	Monday	Tuesday	Wednesday	Thursday	Friday	Saturday
			1	2	3	4
5	6	7	8	9	10	11
12	13	14	15	16	17	18
19	20	21	22	23	24	25
26	27	28				

MEMORY

Make Associations

Use the memory strategy 'Associations' (page 93) to make a connection between an image pair. There are no right answers. Say the association aloud at least 5 times. Move on to the next image pair.

Let's use the example of a nail and a bucket. You can say, 'Nail makes a hole in the Bucket.' Repeat, 'Nail makes hole in bucket. Nail makes hole in bucket.'

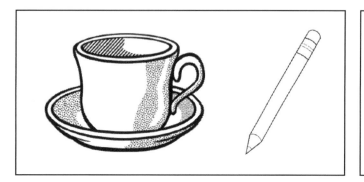
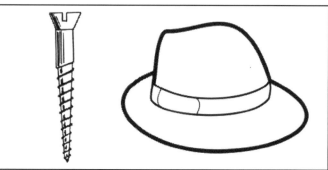
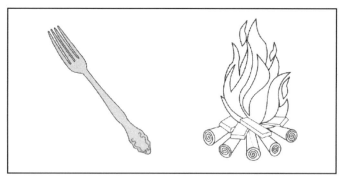
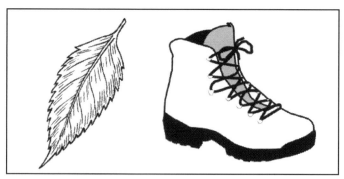
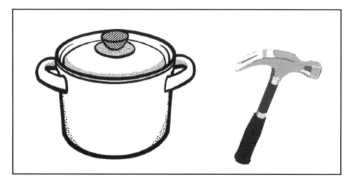
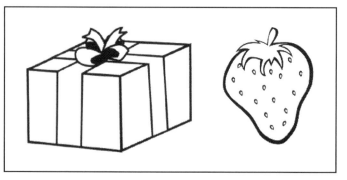

MEMORY

Make Associations

Use the memory strategy 'Associations' (page 93) to make a connection between a word pair. There are no right answers. Say the association aloud at least 5 times. Move on to the next word pair.

Let's use the example of a nail and a bucket. You can say, 'Nail makes a hole in the Bucket.' Repeat, 'Nail makes hole in bucket. Nail makes hole in bucket.'

| Egg | Ball |
| Spoon | Sugar |

| Basket | Salt |
| Tennis | Volcano |

| Door | Candle |
| Vacuum | Boat |

MEMORY

Remembering People's Names

1. Write the name of the person you want to remember: _____

2. Write the same name three more times:

   _____   _____   _____

3. Do you know anyone with that same name? Write down how you know that person. For example: "Jennifer from work" or "Jennifer who lived next door" or "Jennifer who was my daughter's friend."

   _____

   _____

4. Does the name remind you of another word that is easy to picture? For example: Alisha reminds me of "a leash" like a dog leash (silly associations are fine). Write it down.

   _____

   _____

MEMORY

5. Does the name rhyme with another word? Can you make a little "jingle" or "tune" out of the name? For example: Hillary is hilarious. Maria is marvelous. Dave likes to save. Write it down.

_____

_____

6. Which of the previous associations feel "right" to you? The person with the same name? Another word that is easy to picture? Or a rhyming word/jingle? Write the winning association down three more times.

_____

_____

_____

7. Without looking at this paper, say the association aloud three more times.

8. Without looking at this paper, say the name of the person you want to remember.

9. Repeat the association to yourself at least three different times throughout the day. Do this daily for at least one week.

MEMORY

Therapy Team

Use your memory strategies to remember your therapy team's names. First write down their names. Then write down an association for each name (e.g. Dave likes to save).

NURSE. _____

_____

_____

SPEECH THERAPIST. _____

_____

_____

OCCUPATIONAL THERAPIST. _____

_____

_____

PHYSICAL THERAPIST. _____

_____

_____

OTHER TEAM MEMBERS. _____

_____

_____

Names to Pictures

Use your memory strategies to recall the following people's names.

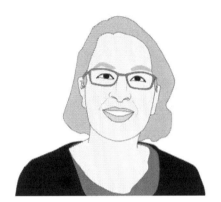
Maria

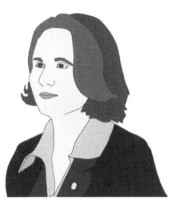
Charlotte

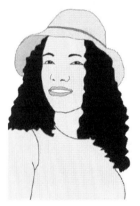
Gigi

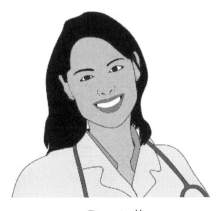
Danielle

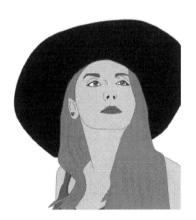
Angela

MEMORY

Page 2 of 2

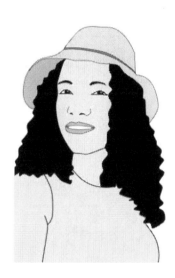
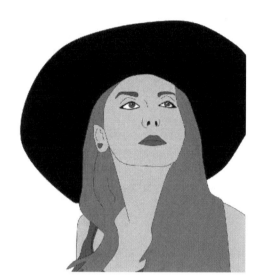
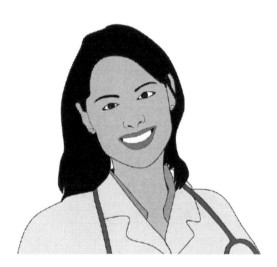
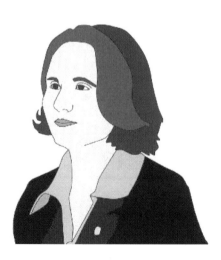
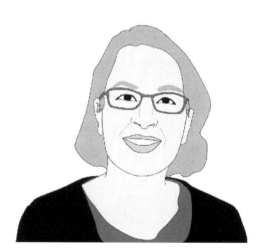

Names to Pictures

Use your memory strategies to recall the following people's names.

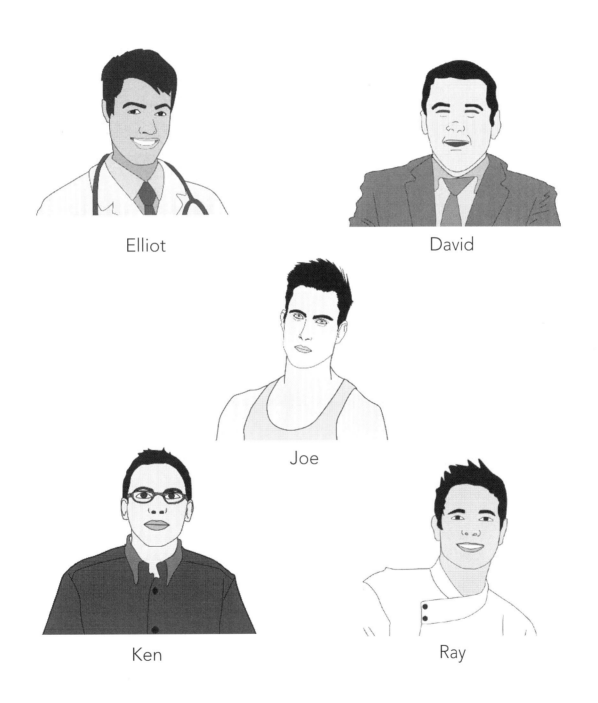

MEMORY

Page 2 of 2

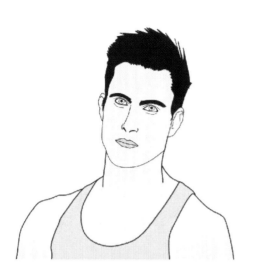
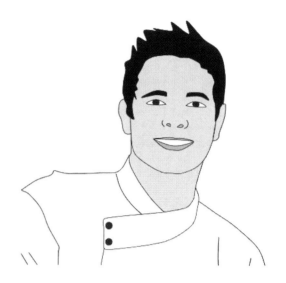
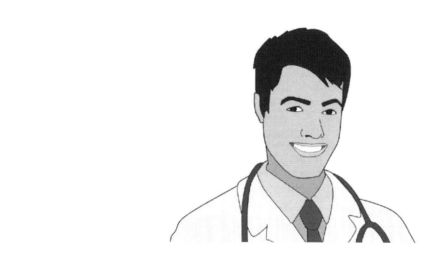
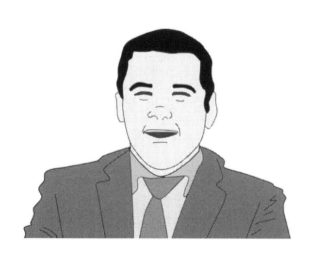
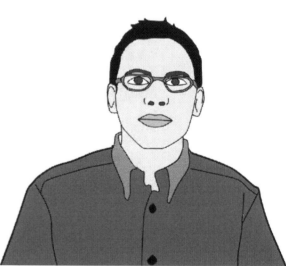

Names to Photos

Use your memory strategies to recall the following people's names.

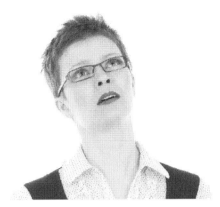
Emily

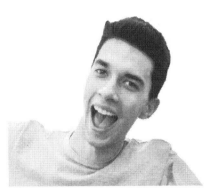
Julian

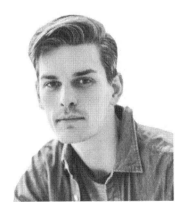
George

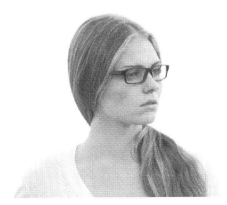
Margaret

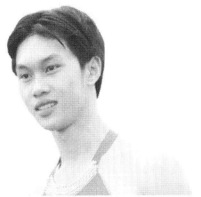
Jin

MEMORY

Page 2 of 2

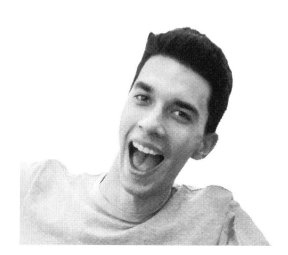
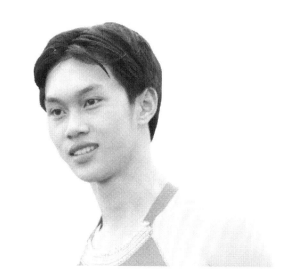
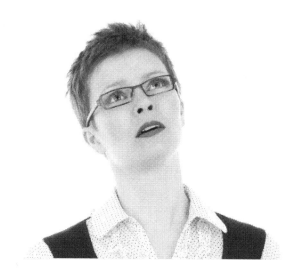
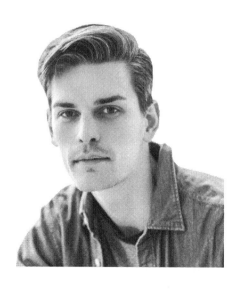
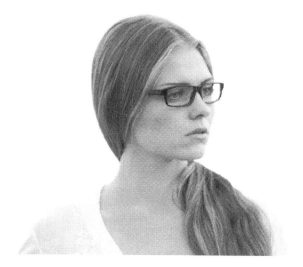

MEMORY

Passwords

To keep your information secure, websites require ever more complex passwords. For example, a password may require at least 8 digits, a capital letter, a symbol, and a number. Use the following tips to create secure passwords and remember/keep track of them.

HOW TO REMEMBER PASSWORDS.
- If you write them down, write them in the same place (e.g. a password notebook). Store it in the same, secure location between uses.
- Use a trusted password manager. Be sure to create an extra-secure password (see tips below) as the master password that unlocks access to your password manager.
- Use mnemonics that are meaningful to you. Use capital and lower case letters, symbols, and acronyms.
- If you can't remember your password, then reset it and use the previous tips to remember the new password in the future.

HOW TO INCREASE SECURITY.
- Combine all of the tips below to create a secure password.
- Make your password as long as possible—8 or more characters.
- Add acronyms: For example, "I love New York" to "ILNY."
- Add alternating capital/lowercase letters: For example, "iLoVeNeWyOrK."
- Replace some letters with numbers/symbols: For example, "p$nNyL@N3."
- Avoid using identifying information that is easy to guess, like birthdays.
- Don't reuse passwords.
- Don't use a single word that can be found in the dictionary of any language.

MEMORY

Group & Memorize

Sort the pictures into different groups. Then, use your memory strategies to memorize each group. Finally, memorize all the items on this page.

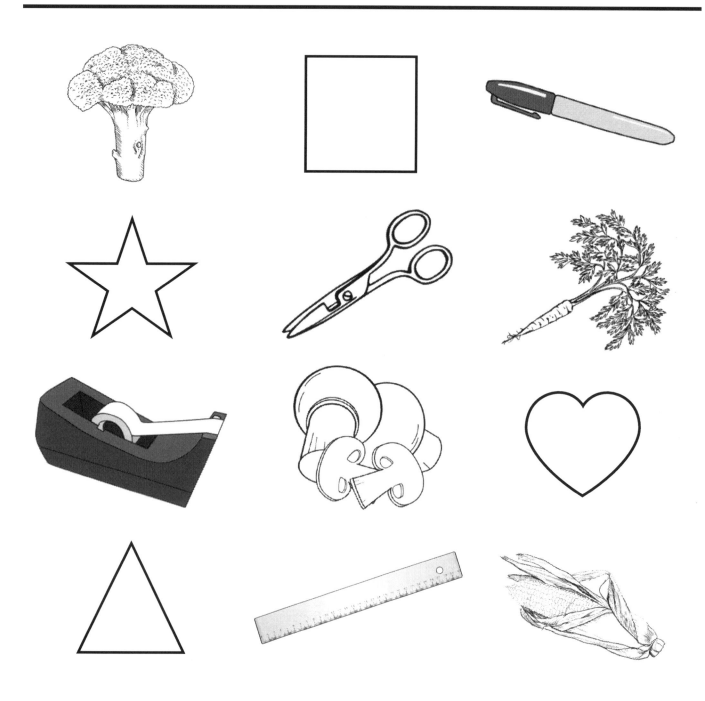

MEMORY

Group & Memorize

Sort the pictures into different groups. Then, use your memory strategies to memorize each group. Finally, memorize all the items on this page.

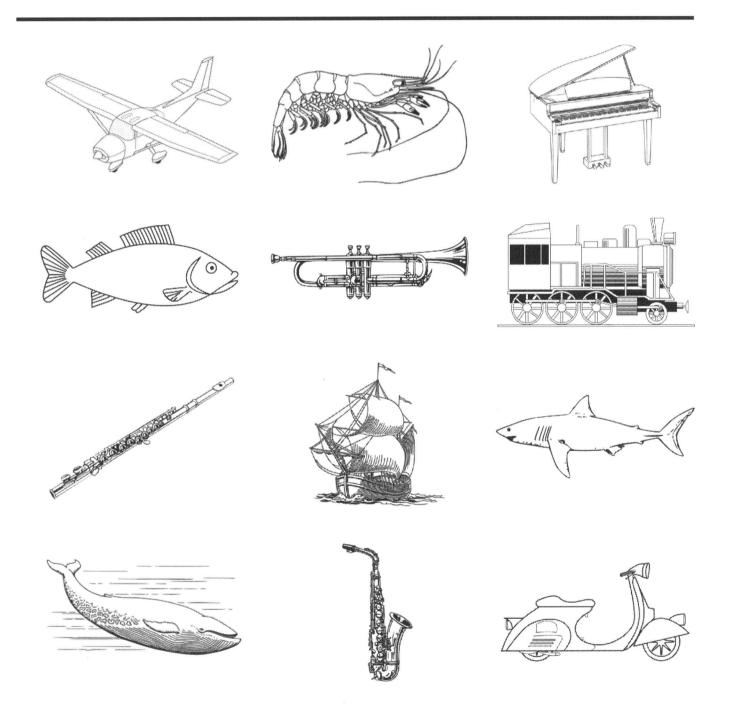

MEMORY

Memorize Lists

WRITE YOUR LIST. Avoid adding extra information.
- A grocery list example: If you always buy whole wheat bread, then just write down "bread."

IDENTIFY GROUPS. There should be at least two groups. Limit groups to 3-5 items each *(Cowan, 2010)*. There can be an "other" group for items that don't quite belong to any specific group.

SORT THE LIST INTO GROUPS. You can do this by rewriting your list. Or highlight each item using a different color for each group (e.g., Dairy is yellow, Produce is green).

READ THE FIRST GROUP ALOUD. Repeat at least three times. Read from your paper as needed.

REPEAT WITHOUT READING. This time, don't look at the paper as you repeat the first group again.
- If you **remembered** all the items, then move on to the next group.
- If you **forgot** one or more items, then read your list aloud at least three times and try again.
- If you're **still having trouble** remembering the items, then try making the groups smaller.

MEMORY

Page 2 of 2

CONTINUE WITH THE OTHER GROUPS. Continue reading aloud and repeating each group until you've memorized the entire list.

REPEAT THE ENTIRE LIST ALOUD. Say your list aloud, group by group.
- If you **remembered** all the items, then repeat the entire list aloud at least three times.
- If you **forgot** one or more items, take a short break then read the list aloud before trying again.

MEMORY

Memorize Lists

Place the items into groups using the blank spaces. Your groups may differ from the spaces provided—that's okay. You can write in the margins as needed. Use your memory strategies to memorize the groups and then the entire list.

GROCERY LIST
- Apples
- Bananas
- Cheese
- Oranges
- Milk
- Half & Half
- Grapes

SHOPPING LIST
- Scissors
- Toilet paper
- Pencils
- Erasers
- Paper plates
- Markers
- Napkins
- Plastic forks

TO DO LIST
- Drop clothes off for donation
- Return blouse
- Buy stamps
- Get the mail
- Buy new blouse
- Buy greeting card

| MEMORY |

Memorize Lists

Place the items into groups using the blank spaces. Your groups may differ from the spaces provided—that's okay. You can write in the margins as needed. Use your memory strategies to memorize the groups and then the entire list.

GROCERY LIST
- Coffee
- Bottled water
- Bread
- Jam
- Juice
- Peanut butter

SHOPPING LIST
- Toothpaste
- Shampoo
- Sponges
- Body wash
- Dish soap
- Conditioner
- Bleach

TO DO LIST
- Call the caterer
- Call the bakery
- Pay rental company deposit
- Check status of refund
- Pay energy bill
- Call bartender

MEMORY

Memorize Lists

Place the items into groups using the blank spaces. Your groups may differ from the spaces provided—that's okay. You can write in the margins as needed. Use your memory strategies to memorize the groups and then the entire list.

GROCERY LIST
- Canned corn
- Milk
- Apples
- Half & half
- Frozen pizza
- Tomatoes
- Lettuce
- Canned tomatoes
- Canned beans
- Ice cream
- Popsicles
- Cheese

SHOPPING LIST
- Nails
- Aluminum foil
- Windshield wipers
- Engine oil
- Plastic wrap
- Screwdriver
- Sandwich bags
- Wiper fluid
- Screws

MEMORY

Memorize Lists

Place the items into groups using the blank spaces. Your groups may differ from the spaces provided—that's okay. You can write in the margins as needed. Use your memory strategies to memorize the groups and then the entire list.

TO DO LIST
- Mow lawn
- Replace windshield wipers
- Plant seeds
- Deposit check
- Water flowers
- Withdraw $60 cash
- Pay water bill
- Pull weeds
- Wash car
- Wax car

GROCERY LIST
- Frozen dinner
- Celery
- Cucumber
- Ice cream
- Flour
- Corn
- Popsicles
- Sugar
- Vanilla flavoring

MEMORY

Memorize Lists

Place the items into groups using the blank spaces. Your groups may differ from the spaces provided—that's okay. You can write in the margins as needed. Use your memory strategies to memorize the groups and then the entire list.

SHOPPING LIST
- Shower curtain
- Bath mat
- Coffee table
- Shower curtain rings
- Armchair
- Area rug
- Hand towel
- Bath towel
- Lamp
- Wall art

TO DO LIST
- Pack bag
- Email client
- Buy school supplies
- Finish work report
- Pick up passport
- Go to PTA meeting
- Buy foreign money
- Drop kids off at mom's house
- Meeting at 10 am

MEMORY

Memorize Lists

Place the items into groups using the blank spaces. Your groups may differ from the spaces provided—that's okay. You can write in the margins as needed. Use your memory strategies to memorize the groups and then the entire list.

GROCERY LIST
- Avocados
- Lemons
- Apples
- Cabbage
- Bell peppers
- Limes
- Oranges
- Grapes
- Carrots
- Grapefruit
- Blueberries
- Bananas

SHOPPING LIST
- Razors
- Colored pencils
- Glue sticks
- Paper towels
- Plastic spoons
- Body wash
- Shaving cream
- Binder
- Ruler
- Toilet paper
- Toothbrush
- Tin foil

MEMORY

Memorize Lists

Place the items into groups using the blank spaces. Your groups may differ from the spaces provided—that's okay. You can write in the margins as needed. Use your memory strategies to memorize the groups and then the entire list.

GROCERY LIST
- Hot dogs
- Lettuce
- Tomatoes
- Sour cream
- Bacon
- Cheese
- Ground beef
- Milk
- Half and Half
- Onions
- Avocados
- Lunch meat

SHOPPING LIST
- Tarp
- Camping chairs
- Diapers
- Pacifier
- Ribbon
- Tape
- Tent
- Baby bottle
- Cooler
- Gift wrap
- Bow
- Baby wipes

> **MEMORY**

Brain Organization Tips

When tackling a multi-step project, use these tips to organize your thoughts and stay on task (Dawson et al., 2009). You can use these tips when preparing for a dinner party, large cleaning project, grocery shopping, or refilling a prescription over the phone.

STOP. Take a break. Ask yourself, "What am I doing?"

GOAL. What's the main task? What are you supposed to be doing?

PLAN. What steps do you need to take to complete the task?

LEARN. Say the steps over and over again.

DO IT! Complete the task.

CHECK. Take a break. Check your work. Ask yourself, "Am I doing what I planned to do?"

MEMORY

Remembering Instructions

Read one instruction aloud, then ask the patient to repeat back the key information. Record accuracy by how many keywords (underlined) the patient recalls. If the patient expresses the main idea in their own words (e.g. they say "go right" for the keywords "turn right"), this counts as accurate.

Go through five instructions, then review the set using the keywords (e.g., "tell me about the garlic" or "what do I combine?")

If patient accuracy is 80% or above: Add five more instructions, then review the entire set of ten instructions, using the keywords. Repeat until accuracy during review falls below 80%.

1. Take <u>tablet</u> <u>twice</u> <u>daily</u>.
2. <u>Preheat</u> <u>oven</u> to <u>450</u> degrees Fahrenheit.
3. Bring <u>photo</u> <u>ID</u> and your <u>insurance card</u>.
4. <u>Stir</u> until <u>mixed</u>.
5. Take a <u>left</u> at the <u>light</u>.
6. Take <u>one</u> <u>pill</u> <u>daily</u> for <u>two</u> <u>weeks</u>.
7. <u>Line up</u> on the <u>right</u> if you <u>prepaid</u>.
8. <u>Enter</u> your <u>phone number</u> and <u>billing address</u>.
9. While <u>pan</u> is <u>heating</u>, <u>mince</u> <u>two</u> <u>cloves of garlic</u>.
10. Take <u>Exit</u> <u>210</u>, then take the <u>first</u> <u>right</u>.

MEMORY

11. Clean the glass and then apply the film.

12. If your last name begins with A through M, go to the left.

13. Park in Lot C, then check in at the Urgent Care desk.

14. Add salt, cinnamon, and nutmeg then mix.

15. Turn left at the red mailbox, then drive another 2 miles.

16. Remove your laptop and take off your shoes and jacket.

17. Push up using your chair's armrests, then stand still.

18. Take 25 mg morning, noon, and night, with water.

19. Go up this elevator to the third floor, then the counter will be on the right.

20. Read the packet, initial each page, and sign on the back.

21. Follow the hallway until it ends, take a left, then the lobby is down the third hallway on the right.

22. Take 1/2 tablet once daily for two weeks, then one tablet daily.

23. Spread cheese mixture on the bottom of a greased 9x13" pan, then top with cooked noodles.

24. In 10 minutes, enter the auditorium using the left-most doors. Your seat will be to the left, in the middle of the row.

25. Insert your debit card, type in your pin number, then press the "Help" button on the bottom-right corner.

> MEMORY

Remembering Appointments

These tips for remembering appointments are simple and effective. But they can take time to become a habit. For one week, try at least one of these tips anytime you need to remember an appointment. Try not to rely on others to remember appointments for you.

BRING A POCKET PLANNER OR CELLPHONE WITH YOU TO APPOINTMENTS. As soon as you schedule a follow-up visit, immediately put the appointment in your planner or cell phone.

DOUBLE CHECK YOUR APPOINTMENTS. When you receive an "appointment reminder" card or call, double check that the appointment is in your calendar, planner, or cellphone.

USE WHITEBOARDS OR MEMO PADS. Place a small magnetic whiteboard or memo pad on your refrigerator. Use it to write down important appointments.

SET ALARMS. Set an alarm for 2 hours before each appointment. Use your alarm clock, cellphone, kitchen timer, or smart speaker to set alarms.

| MEMORY |

Neurology Appointments

Neurologists are medical doctors who treat brain, spinal cord, and nerve issues. They are an important part of the medical team for people with memory and other cognitive challenges.

BEFORE YOUR APPOINTMENT. On the next page, write down:
- **Symptoms**: What are your symptoms? Which is the most concerning?
- **Recent medical history and family history** that relate to neurology
  - *For example, "I had a brain scan in the hospital" or "mom had memory loss."*
- **Questions**: What questions do you have about your symptoms, treatment, or the future?
- **Therapies** you're currently receiving: What are your goals for each therapy?
- **Medications** you're currently taking.

WHAT TO EXPECT AT YOUR APPOINTMENT.
- **Discussion** of your symptoms.
- **A short test or screen** of your cognitive skills.
- **To make a plan**, including follow-up appointments, brain scans, etc.

MEMORY

Appointment Notes

Fill in #1-3 before your appointment. Fill in #4 during your appointment. Date: _____

---

1. SYMPTOMS _____

_____

_____

2. RELEVANT HISTORY _____

_____

_____

3. QUESTIONS _____

_____

_____

_____

4. ANSWERS AND NOTES _____

_____

_____

_____

MEMORY

Page 1 of 4

Memos & Appointments

Use your memory strategies for the exercises below. Read each memo a few times, underlining keywords as you go. Then answer the questions. Try not to look at the memo.

---

1. This is Dina from Dr. Lee's office. I'm calling to confirm your appointment for Friday, January 10th at 8:00 am. Please bring photo ID and your insurance card.
   - What doctor are you meeting?
   - What day is your appointment?
   - What time is your appointment?

2. Hello, my name is Danny, and I'm a physical therapist with Home Health NorthWest. I'm calling to schedule an appointment with you for a physical therapy evaluation. I hope to see you on Thursday at around 10:30 am. Please give me a call back.
   - Who called?
   - What was the name of the company?
   - What time is the appointment?

MEMORY

3. Good morning! Your prescription is ready for pick-up at Main Street Pharmacy. We are open today from 7 am to 6 pm. Please note that if you do not pick up your prescription within 7 days, then it will be re-shelved. Thank you!
- When does the pharmacy close?
- What is the pharmacy's name?
- How many days do you have to pick up the prescription?

4. It has been 3 months since you last visited the chiropractor. Visit us at www.spinewhisperer.com to make a follow-up appointment today!
- When did you last see the chiropractor?
- What is the website?

5. You are now eligible for online check-in. Have your confirmation number ready. Please note that check-in closes 45 minutes prior to boarding time.
- What do you need to have to check-in online?
- When does check-in close?

6. Hi, this is Oliver. I'm a radiology technician at Local Hospital. I received an order for you to complete a swallowing study with us, but I needed some more information before I can schedule the appointment. Please call back at your earliest convenience.
- Who is calling?
- Why is the person calling?

MEMORY

7. This is Bob calling with Healthy Bodies Insurance Company. I have an update about your coverage for your recent stay at the hospital. I can also answer the questions you left on our answering service about outpatient therapy services. I'll try calling back this afternoon.
- What is the name of your health insurance company?
- Why are they calling?

8. Hello, my name is Ashanty, and I'm a speech therapist with Kids Grow Therapy Group. Your usual speech therapist is on vacation, which I believe she told you about, so I will be seeing Emily this week. I'm free on Friday afternoon if that works for you. Please call me back to schedule an appointment. Thanks!
- Who is calling?
- When is she available?
- Where is your usual speech therapist?

9. This is Dr. Goldman from Local Hospital. I reviewed the MRI that you completed yesterday and everything looks good. I don't see any changes from your previous MRI, which is great. If you have any further questions, please call our office anytime.
- Who is calling?
- What type of test did you complete?
- What were the results?

MEMORY

10. Good afternoon. My name is Harold, and I'm calling on behalf of the Census Bureau. Do you have a few minutes to answers five questions about your home? What is your address? Is this home rented or owned? Did you move in during the past 12 months? Has anyone moved in or out of the residence in the past 12 months? And did you complete any construction on the home in the past 12 months? Thank you for your time.
- Who is calling?
- How many questions did he ask?
- What is one question?

MEMORY

Remembering Reading Material

Underline keywords or concepts as you read the following excerpts. After each paragraph, summarize what you just read.

Pride and Prejudice
By Jane Austen

Chapter 1

It is a truth universally acknowledged, that a single man in possession of a good fortune, must be in want of a wife.

However little known the feelings or views of such a man may be on his first entering a neighbourhood, this truth is so well fixed in the minds of the surrounding families, that he is considered the rightful property of some one or other of their daughters.

"My dear Mr. Bennet," said his lady to him one day, "have you heard that Netherfield Park is let at last?"

Mr. Bennet replied that he had not.

"But it is," returned she; "for Mrs. Long has just been here, and she told me all about it." Mr. Bennet made no answer.

"Do you not want to know who has taken it?" cried his wife impatiently.

"You want to tell me, and I have no objection to hearing it."

This was invitation enough.

"Why, my dear, you must know, Mrs. Long says that Netherfield is taken by a young man of large fortune from the north of England; that he came down on Monday in a chaise and four to see the place, and was so much delighted with it, that he agreed with Mr. Morris immediately; that he is to take possession before Michaelmas, and some of his servants are to be in the house by the end of next week."

"What is his name?"

"Bingley."

"Is he married or single?"

"Oh! Single, my dear, to be sure! A single man of large fortune; four or five thousand a year. What a fine thing for our girls!"

"How so? How can it affect them?"

"My dear Mr. Bennet," replied his wife, "how can you be so tiresome! You must know that I am thinking of his marrying one of them."

"Is that his design in settling here?"

"Design! Nonsense, how can you talk so! But it is very likely that he may fall in love with one of them, and therefore you must visit him as soon as he comes."

"I see no occasion for that. You and the girls may go, or you may send them by themselves, which perhaps will be still better, for as you are as handsome as any of them, Mr. Bingley may like you the best of the party."

"My dear, you flatter me. I certainly have had my share of beauty, but I do not pretend to be anything extraordinary now. When a woman has five grown-up daughters, she ought to give over thinking of her own beauty."

"In such cases, a woman has not often much beauty to think of."

"But, my dear, you must indeed go and see Mr. Bingley when he comes into the neighbourhood."

"It is more than I engage for, I assure you."

"But consider your daughters. Only think what an establishment it would be for one of them. Sir William and Lady Lucas are determined to go, merely on that account, for in general, you know, they visit no newcomers. Indeed you must go, for it will be impossible for us to visit him if you do not."

"You are over-scrupulous, surely. I dare say Mr. Bingley will be very glad to see you; and I will send a few lines by you to assure him of my hearty consent to his marrying whichever he chooses of the girls; though I must throw in a good word for my little Lizzy."

"I desire you will do no such thing. Lizzy is not a bit better than the others; and I am sure she is not half so handsome as Jane, nor half so good-humoured as Lydia. But you are always giving her the preference."

"They have none of them much to recommend them," replied he; "they are all silly and ignorant like other girls; but Lizzy has something more of quickness than her sisters."

"Mr. Bennet, how can you abuse your own children in such a way? You take delight in vexing me. You have no compassion for my poor nerves."

"You mistake me, my dear. I have a high respect for your nerves. They are my old friends. I have heard you mention them with consideration these last twenty years at least."

"Ah, you do not know what I suffer."

"But I hope you will get over it, and live to see many young men of four thousand a year come into the neighbourhood."

"It will be no use to us, if twenty such should come, since you will not visit them."

"Depend upon it, my dear, that when there are twenty, I will visit them all."

Mr. Bennet was so odd a mixture of quick parts, sarcastic humour, reserve, and caprice, that the experience of three-and-twenty years had been insufficient to make his wife understand his character. Her mind was less difficult to develop. She was a woman of mean understanding, little information, and uncertain temper. When she was discontented, she fancied herself nervous. The business of her life was to get her daughters married; its solace was visiting and news.

END.

The Adventures of Sherlock Holmes

By Arthur Conan Doyle

"A SCANDAL IN BOHEMIA"

I.

To Sherlock Holmes she is always *the* woman. I have seldom heard him mention her under any other name. In his eyes she eclipses and predominates the whole of her sex. It was not that he felt any emotion akin to love for Irene Adler. All emotions, and that one particularly, were abhorrent to his cold, precise but admirably balanced mind. He was, I take it, the most perfect reasoning and observing machine that the world has seen, but as a lover he would have placed himself in a false position. He never spoke of the softer passions, save with a gibe and a sneer. They were admirable things for the observer—excellent for drawing the veil from men's motives and actions. But for the trained reasoner to admit such intrusions into his own delicate and finely adjusted temperament was to introduce a distracting factor which might throw a doubt upon all his mental results. Grit in a sensitive instrument, or a crack in one of his own high-power lenses, would not be more disturbing than a strong emotion in a nature such as his. And yet there was but one woman to him, and that woman was the late Irene Adler, of dubious and questionable memory.

I had seen little of Holmes lately. My marriage had drifted us away from each other. My own complete happiness, and the home-centred interests which rise up around the man who first finds himself master of his own establishment, were sufficient to absorb all my attention, while Holmes, who loathed every form of society with his whole Bohemian soul, remained in our lodgings in Baker Street, buried among his old books, and alternating from week to week between cocaine and ambition, the drowsiness of the drug, and the fierce energy of his own keen nature. He was still, as ever, deeply attracted by the study of crime, and occupied his immense faculties and extraordinary powers of observation in following out those clues, and clearing up those mysteries which had been abandoned as hopeless by the official police. From time to time I heard some vague account of his doings: of his summons to Odessa in the case of the Trepoff murder, of his clearing up of the singular tragedy of the Atkinson brothers at Trincomalee, and finally of the mission which he had accomplished so delicately and successfully for the reigning family of Holland. Beyond these signs of his activity, however, which I merely shared with all the readers of the daily press, I knew little of my former friend and companion.

One night—it was on the twentieth of March, 1888—I was returning from a journey to a patient (for I had now returned to civil practice), when my way led me through Baker Street. As I passed the well-remembered door, which must always be associated in my mind with my wooing, and with the dark incidents of the Study in Scarlet, I was seized with a keen desire to see Holmes again, and to know how he was employing his extraordinary powers. His rooms were brilliantly lit, and, even as I looked up, I saw his tall, spare figure pass twice in a dark silhouette against the blind. He was pacing the room swiftly, eagerly, with his head sunk upon his chest and his hands clasped behind him. To me, who knew his every mood and habit, his attitude and manner told their own story. He was at work again. He had risen out of his drug-created dreams and was hot upon the scent of some new problem. I rang the bell and was shown up to the chamber which had formerly been in part my own.

His manner was not effusive. It seldom was; but he was glad, I think, to see me. With hardly a word spoken, but with a kindly eye, he waved me to an armchair, threw across his case of cigars, and indicated a spirit case and a gasogene in the corner. Then he stood before the fire and looked me over in his singular introspective fashion.

"Wedlock suits you," he remarked. "I think, Watson, that you have put on seven and a half pounds since I saw you."

"Seven!" I answered.

"Indeed, I should have thought a little more. Just a trifle more, I fancy, Watson. And in practice again, I observe. You did not tell me that you intended to go into harness."

"Then, how do you know?"

"I see it, I deduce it. How do I know that you have been getting yourself very wet lately, and that you have a most clumsy and careless servant girl?"

"My dear Holmes," said I, "this is too much. You would certainly have been burned, had you lived a few centuries ago. It is true that I had a country walk on Thursday and came home in a dreadful mess, but as I have changed my clothes I can't imagine how you deduce it. As to Mary Jane, she is incorrigible, and my wife has given her notice, but there, again, I fail to see how you work it out."

He chuckled to himself and rubbed his long, nervous hands together.

"It is simplicity itself," said he; "my eyes tell me that on the inside of your left shoe, just where the firelight strikes it, the leather is scored by six almost parallel cuts. Obviously they have been caused by someone who has very carelessly scraped round the edges of the sole in order to remove crusted mud from it. Hence, you see, my double deduction that you had been out in vile weather, and that you had a particularly malignant boot-slitting specimen of the London slavey. As to your practice, if a gentleman walks into my rooms smelling of iodoform, with a black mark of nitrate of silver upon his right forefinger, and a bulge on the right side of his top-hat to show where he has secreted his stethoscope, I must be dull, indeed, if I do not pronounce him to be an active member of the medical profession."

I could not help laughing at the ease with which he explained his process of deduction. "When I hear you give your reasons," I remarked, "the thing always appears to me to be so ridiculously simple that I could easily do it myself, though at each successive instance of your reasoning I am baffled until you explain your process. And yet I believe that my eyes are as good as yours."

END.

Momotaro, or The Story of the Son of a Peach

*"Japanese Fairy Tales"
Complied by
Yei Theodora Ozaki*

Long, long ago there lived, an old man and an old woman; they were peasants, and had to work hard to earn their daily rice. The old man used to go and cut grass for the farmers around, and while he was gone the old woman, his wife, did the work of the house and worked in their own little rice field.

One day the old man went to the hills as usual to cut grass and the old woman took some clothes to the river to wash.

It was nearly summer, and the country was very beautiful to see in its fresh greenness as the two old people went on their way to work. The grass on the banks of the river looked like emerald velvet, and the pussy willows along the edge of the water were shaking out their soft tassels.

The breezes blew and ruffled the smooth surface of the water into wavelets, and passing on touched the cheeks of the old couple who, for some reason they could not explain, felt very happy that morning.

The old woman at last found a nice spot by the river bank and put her basket down. Then she set to work to wash the clothes; she took them one by one out of the basket and washed them in the river and rubbed them on the stones. The water was as clear as crystal, and she could see the tiny fish swimming to and fro, and the pebbles at the bottom.

As she was busy washing her clothes a great peach came bumping down the stream. The old woman looked up from her work and saw this large peach. She was sixty years of age, yet in all her life she had never seen such a big peach as this.

"How delicious that peach must be!" she said to herself. "I must certainly get it and take it home to my old man."

She stretched out her arm to try and get it, but it was quite out of her reach. She looked about for a stick, but there was not one to be seen, and if she went to look for one she would lose the peach.

Stopping a moment to think what she would do, she remembered an old charm-verse. Now she began to clap her hands to keep time to the rolling of the peach down stream, and while she clapped she sang this song:

*"Distant water is bitter,
The near water is sweet;
Pass by the distant water
And come into the sweet."*

Strange to say, as soon as she began to repeat this little song the peach began to come nearer and nearer the bank where the old woman was standing, till at last it stopped just in front of her so that she was able to take it up in her hands. The old woman was delighted. She could not go on with her work, so happy and excited was she, so she put all the clothes back in her bamboo basket, and with the basket on her back and the peach in her hand she hurried homewards.

It seemed a very long time to her to wait till her husband returned. The old man at last came back as the sun was setting, with a big bundle of grass on his back—so big that he was almost hidden and she could hardly see him. He seemed very tired and used the scythe for a walking stick, leaning on it as he walked along.

As soon as the old woman saw him she called out:

"O Fii San! (old man) I have been waiting for you to come home for such a long time to-day!"

"What is the matter? Why are you so impatient?" asked the old man, wondering at her unusual eagerness. "Has anything happened while I have been away?"

"Oh, no!" answered the old woman, "nothing has happened, only I have found a nice present for you!"

"That is good," said the old man. He then washed his feet in a basin of water and stepped up to the veranda.

The old woman now ran into the little room and brought out from the cupboard the big peach. It felt even heavier than before. She held it up to him, saying:

"Just look at this! Did you ever see such a large peach in all your life?"

When the old man looked at the peach he was greatly astonished and said:

"This is indeed the largest peach I have ever seen! Wherever did you buy it?"

"I did not buy it," answered the old woman. "I found it in the river where I was washing." And she told him the whole story.

"I am very glad that you have found it. Let us eat it now, for I am hungry," said the O Fii San.

He brought out the kitchen knife, and, placing the peach on a board, was about to cut it when, wonderful to tell, the peach split in two of itself and a clear voice said:

"Wait a bit, old man!" and out stepped a beautiful little child.

The old man and his wife were both so astonished at what they saw that they fell to the ground. The child spoke again:

"Don't be afraid. I am no demon or fairy. I will tell you the truth. Heaven has had compassion on you. Every day and every night you have lamented that you had no child. Your cry has been heard and I am sent to be the son of your old age!"

On hearing this the old man and his wife were very happy. They had cried night and day for sorrow at having no child to help them in their lonely old age, and now that their prayer was answered they were so lost with joy that they did not know where to put their hands or their feet. First the old man took the child up in his arms, and then the old woman did the same; and they named him MOMOTARO, OR SON OF A PEACH, because he had come out of a peach.

END.

The Story of Ali Baba and the Forty Thieves.

"The Arabian Nights: Their Best-Known Tales"
Edited by Kate Douglas Wiggin & Nora A. Smith.

In a town in Persia, there lived two brothers, one named Cassim, the other Ali Baba. Their father left them scarcely anything; but as he had divided his little property equally between them, it would seem that their fortune ought to have been equal; but chance determined otherwise.

Cassim married a wife, who soon after became heiress to a large sum, and to a warehouse full of rich goods; so that he all at once became one of the richest and most considerable merchants, and lived at his ease. Ali Baba, on the other hand, who had married a woman as poor as himself, lived in a very wretched habitation, and had no other means to maintain his wife and children but his daily labour of cutting wood, and bringing it to town to sell, upon three asses, which were his whole substance.

One day, when Ali Baba was in the forest, and had just cut wood enough to load his asses, he saw at a distance a great cloud of dust, which seemed to be driven toward him: he observed it very attentively, and distinguished soon after a body of horse. Though there had been no rumour of robbers in that country, Ali Baba began to think that they might prove such, and without considering what might become of his asses, was resolved to save himself. He climbed up a large, thick tree, whose branches, at a little distance from the ground, were so close to one another that there was but little space between them. He placed himself in the middle, from whence he could see all that passed without being discovered; and the tree stood at the base of a single rock, so steep and craggy that nobody could climb up it.

The troop, who were all well mounted and armed, came to the foot of this rock, and there dismounted. Ali Baba counted forty of them, and, from their looks and equipage, was assured that they were robbers. Nor was he mistaken in his opinion; for they were a troop of banditti, who, without doing any harm to the neighbourhood, robbed at a distance, and made that place their rendezvous; but what confirmed him in his opinion was, that every man unbridled his horse, tied him to some shrub, and hung about his neck a bag of corn which they brought behind them. Then each of them took his saddle wallet, which seemed to Ali Baba to be full of gold and silver from its weight. One, who was the most personable amongst them, and whom he took to be their captain, came with his wallet on his back under the tree in which Ali Baba was concealed, and making his way through some shrubs, pronounced these words so distinctly: "Open, Sesame," that Ali Baba heard him. As soon as the captain of the robbers had uttered these words, a door opened in the rock; and after he had made all his troop enter before him, he followed them, when the door shut again of itself. The robbers stayed some time within the rock, and Ali Baba, who feared that some one, or all of them together, might come out and catch him, if he should endeavour to make his escape, was obliged to sit patiently in the tree. He was nevertheless tempted to get down, mount one of their horses, and lead another, driving his asses before him with all the haste he could to town; but the uncertainty of the event made him choose the safest course.

At last the door opened again, and the forty robbers came out. As the captain went in last, he came out first, and stood to see them all pass by him, when Ali Baba heard him make the door close by pronouncing these words: "Shut, Sesame." Every man went and bridled his horse, fastened his wallet, and mounted again; and when the captain saw them all ready, he put himself at their head, and they returned the way they had come. Ali Baba did not immediately quit his tree; for, said he to himself, they may have forgotten something and may come back again, and then I shall be taken. He followed them with his eyes as far as he could see them; and afterward stayed a considerable time before he descended. Remembering the words the captain of the robbers used to cause the door to open and shut, he had the curiosity to try if his pronouncing them would have the same effect. Accordingly, he went among the shrubs, and perceiving the door concealed behind them, stood before it, and said: "Open, Sesame!" The door instantly flew wide open. Ali Baba, who expected a dark dismal cavern, was surprised to see it well lighted and spacious, in the form of a vault, which received the light from an opening at the top of the rock. He saw all sorts of provisions, rich bales of silk stuff, brocade, and valuable carpeting, piled upon one another; gold and silver ingots in great heaps, and money in bags. The sight of all these riches made him suppose that this cave must have been occupied for ages by robbers, who had succeeded one another. Ali Baba did not stand long to consider what he should do, but went immediately into the cave, and as soon as he had entered, the door shut of itself, but this did not disturb him, because he knew the secret to open it again. He never regarded the silver, but made the best use of his time in carrying out as much of the gold coin as he thought his three asses could carry. He collected his asses, which were dispersed, and when he had loaded them with the bags, laid wood over in such a manner that they could not be seen. When he had done he stood before the door, and pronouncing the words: "Shut, Sesame!" the door closed after him, for it had shut of itself while he was within, but remained open while he was out. He then made the best of his way to town.

END.

PROBLEM SOLVING

Problem solving is the cognitive process of identifying and coming up with solutions to difficult issues. The goal of treatment is to improve problem solving skills and/or compensate for deficits in order to increase independence, safety, and quality of life. Choose problem solving goals and techniques based on the patient's previous and current levels of functioning, amount of support available, motivation, insight into deficits, and other factors.

Problem solving treatment includes:
- Restorative treatment (e.g. improved learning)
- Compensatory treatment (e.g. changes to the home)

PROBLEM SOLVING

Therapist Instructions

EVALUATIONS.
- Cognitive screens include the *MoCA*, *MMSE*, and *SLUMS*.
- Formal batteries include the *Delis-Kaplan Executive Function System* (D-KEFS), parts of the *Wechsler Adult Intelligence Scale* (WAIS-IV), *Rey–Osterrieth Complex Figure Test*, and *Dysexecutive Questionnaire*.
- Informal cognitive-linguistic evaluations often include questions about basic safety (e.g., using call lights, calling 911), simple math, making inferences, and interpreting reading material (e.g. medication labels).

DAY ONE OF TREATMENT. Provide the following handouts, as needed:
- Homework Log, Monthly Calendar, Impairments, Complications After a Stroke, neuroanatomy illustrations, Medication Organization, Organize Your Bills, Medical Alert Systems, Avoiding Falls, Low Vision Tips, Hearing Aids Care, Medical Team Phone Numbers, Meal Planning
- Highlight key points on the handouts, then review with your patients. Ask questions to make sure they understand the content. Answer any questions they may have.

FOR THERAPIST EYES ONLY. Therapist treatment guides are marked with a gray background or header. Some caregivers and patients may benefit from having a copy.
- Task Analysis, TEACH-M, and Making Modifications

STRATEGIES. Review the selected strategies, provide a model, then ask for return demonstrations.
- Filling a Pill Box, Setting Goals, My Goals, Organize Your Bills, Avoiding Falls, Smart Speakers, Low Vision Tips, Hearing Aids Care, Meal Planning

PROBLEM SOLVING

COMPLICATIONS AFTER A STROKE (PAGE 187). This handout can help many of our patients, not just those with problem solving difficulties.
- Use the brain illustrations that follow to educate about brain damage and neuroplasticity.

FILLING A PILL BOX (PAGE 192). Have this out as you practice filling a pill box with your patient.
- If you're not in the patient's home, then practice this task using a weekly pill box with easy press tabs (found at most big-box stores and pharmacies) and beads.

SETTING GOALS (PAGES 193). Making and reaching personal goals can improve confidence, independence, and quality of life.
- Having personal goals can help patients feel a sense of agency as they navigate major changes to their health and lifestyle.
- It may take several weeks for patients to make goals and create a plan to achieve them. Use the worksheets to gradually develop the patient's goals.
- Use with the My Goals handout (page 194), Daily Schedule worksheet (page 119), and Monthly Calendar handout (page 121).

SMART SPEAKERS (PAGE 199). For patients with an Amazon Echo or similar smart-speaker. Review these skills with the patient, provide models, and ask for return demonstrations.

REVIEW WITH A CAREGIVER. The Medical Alert Systems (pages 197), Low Vision Tips (page 200), Hearing Aids Care (page 201), and Emergency Plan (page 210).

SEQUENCING (PAGES 211). These worksheets can be used to segue into practical sequencing tasks, such as making a cup of tea or making the bed. Increase complexity by asking the patient to name the task (e.g. "sending a letter").

PROBLEM SOLVING

MEAL PLANNING WORKSHEETS (PAGES 218). For patients who want to be more independent with meal preparation.
- Treatment order: Review the Meal Planning worksheet, then the Meals this Week worksheet, and finally the Groceries for Meals and Grocery List worksheets.

BALANCE A CHECKBOOK (PAGES 222). Use these worksheets if your patient uses a checkbook or is up for a more complex math challenge.

MATH TASKS. The patient may use a calculator and paper and pen as needed for any of the math worksheets, including Practical Math (page 202), Balance a Checkbook, and Everyday Math (page 228).

THINGS TO THINK ABOUT.
- Dates are abbreviated in the American format of MM/DD/YY.
- Some tasks include two pages. Print one-sided (so the patient doesn't need to flip the paper back and forth).
- Your goal is for the patient to return to their previous level of functioning, or as close to it as possible.
    - Choose tasks that are relevant and practical to the patient. For example, if your patient used a calculator before her stroke to balance a checkbook, then she should continue using a calculator.
    - Help your patient identify their problem solving goals, and focus on the top 1-3 issues.

PROBLEM SOLVING

Contents

Task Analysis………………………………	183
TEACH-M…………………………………..	184
Making Modifications………………………	185
Impairments…………………………………	186
Complications After a Stroke………………	187
Neuroanatomy & Physiology Illustrations…	189
Medication Organization…………………	191
Filling a Pill Box……………………………	192
Setting Goals………………………………	193
My Goals………………………………	194
Two-Week Goal……………….…………	195
Organize Your Bills………………………..	196
Medical Alert Systems……………………	197
Avoiding Falls………………………………	198
Smart Speakers……………………………	199
Low Vision Tips……………………………	200
Hearing Aids Care…………………………	201
Practical Math……..………………………	202
Math in Everyday Life……………………	208
Medical Team Phone Numbers…………	209
Emergency Plan……………………………	210
Sequencing…………………………………	211
Make a Schedule…………………………	215
Meal Planning……………………………..	218
Meals This Week………………..………	219
Groceries for Meals……………………	220
Grocery List *(by category)*…………..	221

PROBLEM SOLVING

    Balance a Checkbook……….................…..   222
    Everyday Math…….....………………………   228

SEE ALSO

        Neuroplasticity………………………..   24
        Daily Schedule……………………….   119
        Brain Organization Tips……………..   155

PROBLEM SOLVING

Task Analysis

Task analysis helps patients learn new skills by breaking down a task into smaller steps (Sohlberg et al., 2005). For example, 'Checking and Deleting Voicemails' can be broken down into these steps: "Touch the phone icon, touch the voicemail button, touch play," and so on. Task analysis is especially handy when working on more complex tasks. Use task analysis to:

- Check blood sugar levels
- Transfer from a wheelchair
- Manage oxygen tubing
- Set up automatic payments for recurring bills
- Plan trips to the grocery store
- Prepare for a dinner party
- Refill a prescription over the phone
- Set an alarm on a smart speaker or cell phone
- Play a movie on *Netflix™*
- Read and delete emails
- Buy items online
- Make a hair salon appointment over the phone
- Use Self Checkout at the store
- Look up the weather forecast online
- Check store hours and phone numbers online
- Set a timer on your oven
- Listen to and delete voicemails
- Use *Google Maps™* to find a local store

PROBLEM SOLVING

TEACH-M

TEACH-M is an acronym for 6 ways to learn new skills (Ehlhardt et al., 2005). Use TEACH-M to help your patients increase independence with daily tasks (e.g. medication management).

TASK ANALYSIS. Help your patient break down the task into smaller steps.

ERRORLESS LEARNING. Focus on accuracy throughout the task. Emphasize not guessing. Minimize guessing by giving enough help (e.g. verbal cues to double check the medication labels).

ASSESS PERFORMANCE. Teach your patient to check their accuracy after each step of the task.

CUMULATIVE REVIEW. Have your patient repeat all the steps of the entire task. Then review how they did on the entire task.

HIGH NUMBER OF PRACTICE TRIALS. Have your patient complete the entire task over and over again.

METACOGNITION. Help patients improve awareness about how they perform on a task.
- Before the task, ask the patient to predict how they'll do.
- After the task, ask them to assess how they did.
- Discuss how their assessment of their own performance compares with how they actually did on the task.

PROBLEM SOLVING

Making Modifications

Modifications to a patient's environment or tasks can improve problem solving skills. They can also help patients compensate for deficits.

ADAPT THE ENVIRONMENT.
- **Reduce clutter**: take down extraneous wall art, donate or store unnecessary items (e.g., old papers, excess furniture)
- **Remove distractions**: reduce excess noise and visual distractions (e.g., turn off the TV, shut the door)
- **Organize the space**: assign specific places for specific things (e.g. keys go in the bowl by the front door)

MODIFY THE TASK. Make tasks easier.
- **Provide cues and prompts**
- **Use task analysis** (break down tasks into smaller, simpler steps)
- **Identify other factors** that may be impacting the patient's ability to problem solve
    - Physiological factors include issues with sleep, nutrition, medication side effects, pain, comorbidities, etc. *(National Institute on Aging, 2020)*
    - Psychological factors include depression and stress
    - Reach out to the patient's physician or nurse for more information

PROBLEM SOLVING

Impairments

Common problem solving impairments include difficulty with the following:

EXECUTIVE FUNCTIONING. Executive functions help you plan, organize, problem solve, and correct errors. An impairment can make it harder to complete everyday tasks, learn new things, and solve problems.

AWARENESS. Difficulty with being aware of your strengths, weaknesses, and when you need help.

ORGANIZATION. Difficulty with creating structure and organizing information.

GENERATIVE THINKING. Difficulty with creating new ideas or coming up with different ways to accomplish a goal.

INITIATION. Difficulty with starting a task.

MOTIVATION. Difficulty with the drive to start and complete a task.

INHIBITION. Difficulty with stopping yourself from acting on impulse.

PERSISTENCE. Difficulty with the resolve and commitment to continue with a task.

> **PROBLEM SOLVING**

Complications After a Stroke

The following are potentially dangerous complications after a stroke or brain injury. Contact your doctor if you experience any concerning symptoms or have other concerns.

FATIGUE. Due to sleeping poorly, poor nutrition, weakness, not enough exercise, and medication side effects.

DEPRESSION AND ANXIETY. Very common after stroke or brain injury due to sudden life changes.

SHOULDER PAIN. Due to muscle weakness or paralysis.

URINARY TRACT INFECTION. Due to reduced bladder control *(American Heart Association, 2015)*.

HEADACHES. Possibly a side effect of new medications or fatigue *(Stroke Association, n.d.)*

PNEUMONIA. Infection of the lungs due to reduced mobility or aspiration.

RECURRENT STROKES. Having another stroke. Risk factors for having another stroke include hypertension, diabetes, sleep apnea, and tobacco and alcohol use. Talk with your doctor about how to reduce your risk *(Oza et al., 2017)*.

PROBLEM SOLVING

PRESSURE ULCERS. Bedsores due to reduced mobility.

CONTRACTURES. Shortened, tight muscles due in part to reduced mobility and lack of movement.

SEIZURES. Due to changes in electrical activity in your brain after a stroke or brain injury.

HIGH BLOOD PRESSURE. Due to stress, elevated brain pressure, or pain.

BRAIN EDEMA. Swelling of the brain; a serious condition that can be caused by brain injury.

DEEP VEIN THROMBOSIS. Blood clots, usually in the leg, due to reduced mobility.

PROBLEM SOLVING

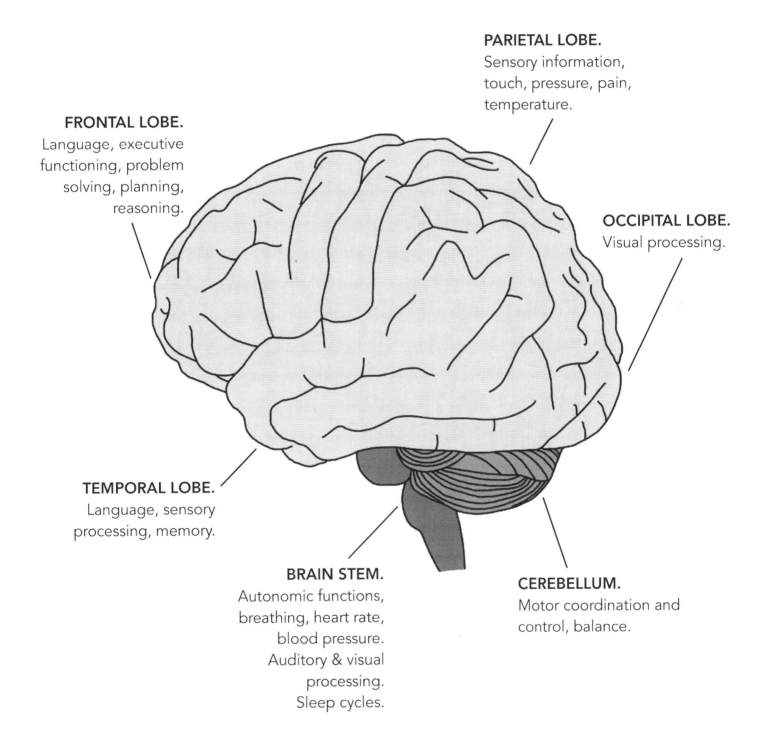

FRONTAL LOBE. Language, executive functioning, problem solving, planning, reasoning.

PARIETAL LOBE. Sensory information, touch, pressure, pain, temperature.

OCCIPITAL LOBE. Visual processing.

TEMPORAL LOBE. Language, sensory processing, memory.

BRAIN STEM. Autonomic functions, breathing, heart rate, blood pressure. Auditory & visual processing. Sleep cycles.

CEREBELLUM. Motor coordination and control, balance.

PROBLEM SOLVING

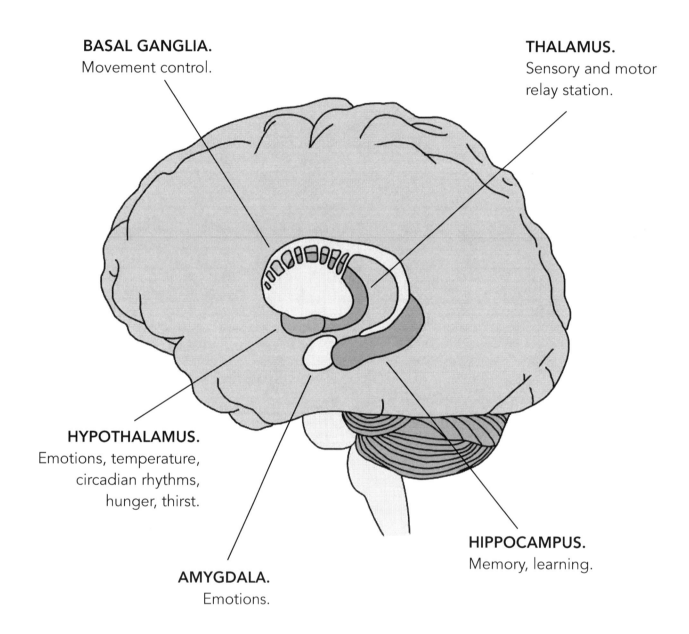

> PROBLEM SOLVING

Medication Organization

Keeping your medications organized is important for your health and safety. Speak with your pharmacist or nurse for more information.

PRESORTED PACKS.
- Your pharmacy can place all of your medications into bubble packs. This replaces the need for a pill box. But be aware that the extra service cost may not be covered by your insurance.
- Amazon.com's *PillPack™* is a free service that sorts your medications and supplements into small plastic packs. Most insurance companies are accepted. Search "Amazon Pharmacy" online for more information.

DISPENSERS. Automatic pill dispensers are usually large, round pill boxes that are locked. They allow access to your medications only at pre-set times. An alarm will sound at those times. A popular dispenser manufacturer is *MedReady™*.

MAIL-IN. Your medications can be mailed to your house so you don't need to call and travel to the pharmacy. Contact your insurance company to see if you are eligible.

ALARMS. Use a cellphone or a smart speaker device (e.g. Amazon Echo) to set repeating alarms every time you need to take or order your medications.

> **PROBLEM SOLVING**

Filling a Pill Box

Fill out your pill box at the same time and day every week. Turn off the TV, silence your cellphone, and avoid having conversations while filling out your pill box. See pages 116 and 191 for more ways to organize your medications.

---

1. Place all of your prescription bottles on the **left side** of the table.

2. **Open up** all the compartments in the pill box.

3. Take **one prescription bottle** and fill in one week's worth.

4. **Double check** your work.

5. Place the bottle to the **right side** of the table.

6. Complete steps 3 - 5 for the rest of your prescriptions.

PROBLEM SOLVING

Setting Goals

WHAT IS YOUR NORMAL ROUTINE? Walk me through a normal day. Now walk me through what a normal day used to look like.

WHAT IS MISSING? List the things that you used to do that you would like to do again (these will become your goals).

WHAT IS REASONABLE IN THE SHORT TERM? Given your new challenges, which of these goals can you get back to in the next two weeks? You may need to make your goal easier, and that's okay. You can gradually work towards any bigger goals.

CHANGE YOUR ROUTINE. What could you do tomorrow to reach your goal? What 1-3 steps can you take this week to reach you goal? How would your routine change?

MAKE A SCHEDULE. On the next page, write down your current and previous routines (steps 1 and 2). Add your 2-week goal (step 3). Now, add the steps you will take to reach this goal (step 4).
- *For example, your goal is to walk 3 days per week. But it's not yet safe for you to walk alone. To your schedule, add, "Ask a friend to walk with me on Mondays, Wednesdays, and Fridays after dinner."*

REPEAT. Repeat the steps for all of your goals.

My Goals

Page 2 of 3

1. CURRENT ROUTINE.

Morning _____

_____

_____

_____

Noon _____

_____

_____

_____

Evening _____

_____

_____

_____

2. PREVIOUS ROUTINE.

Morning _____

_____

_____

_____

Noon _____

_____

_____

_____

Evening _____

_____

_____

_____

3. TWO-WEEK GOAL.

Circle activities from your previous routine that are missing from your current routine. Which of these could you add within two weeks?

_____

4. MAKE A NEW SCHEDULE.

Add steps toward your goal to your daily schedule (next page).

TWO-WEEK GOAL:

Write down the steps you can take to reach your goal.

SUNDAY	MONDAY	TUESDAY	WEDNESDAY	THURSDAY	FRIDAY	SATURDAY
Week 1						
Week 2						

PROBLEM SOLVING

Organize Your Bills

GET ORGANIZED. Make a list of all of your bills. Choose a specific place to put your bills as soon as they arrive (e.g., a basket or brightly colored folder).

KEEP A PHONE/WEBSITE LIST. Keep a list of important phone numbers and/or websites, including Customer Support lines for credit cards and banks.

STICK TO A SCHEDULE. Mark the due dates on your calendar for every month. Decide when to pay your bills every month (end of the month, mid-month, or both).

USE AUTOMATIC PAYMENTS. Set up automatic payments for your recurring bills (e.g., utilities, credit cards).

> PROBLEM SOLVING

Medical Alert Systems

These are devices that you wear in case of a medical emergency. When activated, some systems will call a pre-programmed contact, such as a relative. Other systems will call a 24/7 dispatch center for a monthly cost.

POPULAR MEDICAL ALERT SYSTEMS.
- *Medical Guardian™*
- *Life Alert®*
- *GreatCall®*
- *Alert-1®*
- *LifeStation®*
- *Bay Alarm Medical®*
- *Philips Lifeline®*
- *MobileHelp®*

> PROBLEM SOLVING

Avoiding Falls

As we age, we become more susceptible to falls. Falls can cause serious injuries, including broken bones and traumatic brain injuries. Falls can also lead to frailty, less physical activity, and even a higher risk of death (Centers for Disease Control and Prevention, 2020). *But there is plenty you can do to reduce your risk of falls!*

REVIEW YOUR MEDICATIONS. Some medications can cause drowsiness or dizziness, which may increase your risk for falls. Speak with your doctor.

GET YOUR EYES & EARS CHECKED. Order new prescription lenses or hearing aids as needed (National Institute on Aging, 2017b).

IMPROVE YOUR STRENGTH. Complete your physical and occupational therapy exercises. Plan a regular exercise program that's right for you. Regular exercise makes you stronger and more flexible.

IMPROVE YOUR BALANCE. Physical therapy exercises, yoga, and tai chi can help with balance.

USE ASSISTIVE DEVICES. Use a cane, walker, wheelchair, and grab bars as recommended.

MODIFY YOUR HOME. Remove rugs, add in more and brighter lights, get rid of clutter. Visit the National Institute on Aging's website for more information about Fall-Proofing Your Home (National Institute on Aging, 2017).

> **PROBLEM SOLVING**

Smart Speakers

Smart speakers, like the Amazon Echo "Alexa" device, can help with the following:

ALARMS. "Set an alarm for 7 am everyday" or "Set an alarm for 4 pm every Monday, Wednesday, and Friday."

TIMERS. "Set a 5 minute timer."

REMINDERS. "Remind me to go to the post office today at noon" or "Add bread to my shopping list."

CALENDAR. "Add a doctor's appointment to my calendar on May 21st at 10 am" or "When does spring begin?"

SPELLING. "How do you spell 'dysphagia'?" or "How do you pronounce 'o-r-e-g-o-n'?"

CALCULATIONS. "What's 365 times 50?"

CONVERSIONS. "How many tablespoons is 3 cups?"

PROBLEM SOLVING

Low Vision Tips

REMOVE CLUTTER, CORDS, AND THROW RUGS. Helps avoid falls and bumping into objects.

ADD LIGHTS. Add overhead lights throughout the house to reduce shadows and flexible lamps for reading *(The American Occupational Therapy Association, 2013)*.

GET ORGANIZED. Organize important papers in different colored containers or folders. Organize your refrigerator to easily find foods (e.g. by type of food). Use drawer dividers or containers to organize toiletries, tools, etc. Use large labels.

USE CONTRASTS. Objects will stand out if placed on a contrasting color.
- *For example, choose a dark grab bar for a white wall, or a dark bathmat with rubber grips on a light-colored floor.*

GET DIGITAL. Increase font size and contrast on your computer, tablet, or smartphone.

LISTEN TO AUDIOBOOKS. You can purchase audiobooks or borrow them for free through your library.
- Download **Libby™**, a free app that connects to your library account to check out eBooks and audiobooks.

> **PROBLEM SOLVING**

Hearing Aids Care

Wear your hearing aids as recommended by your audiologist, including during therapy sessions and appointments. Regular maintenance can help avoid common issues.

INSPECT THE OUTSIDE CASING. Check for cracks or chips. Contact your audiologist or hearing aid center for more information.

KEEP THE BATTERY DOOR CLOSED. Apply light pressure to the door.

CHECK THE MICROPHONE. Place the hearing aid in your ear and lightly brush it. If you hear a scratchy sound, then the microphone is working *(Banks, 2020)*.

CLEAN DAILY. With a hearing aid cleaning brush or very soft toothbrush (dry and clean), gently brush the entire cover. Then wipe with a soft towel.

CLEAN WEEKLY. Use a wax pick to remove wax buildup (but do not pick around the microphone).

MAINTAIN BATTERIES. Clean battery compartments regularly with the brush. Replace or charge batteries often.

PROBLEM SOLVING

Practical Math

Use a calculator and pen and paper as needed.

CALCULATING DISCOUNTS. What is your price after the discount?

1. 50% off of a $20 item _____

2. 10% off of a $10 item _____

3. 20% off of a $10 item _____

4. 30% off of a $100 item _____

5. 25% off of a $1,000 item _____

6. 40% off of a $100 item _____

7. 60% off of a $60 item _____

8. 30% off of a $30 item _____

9. 40% off of a $50 item _____

10. 75% off of a $60 item _____

PROBLEM SOLVING

Practical Math

Use a calculator and pen and paper as needed.

CALCULATING TOTALS. What is your total price for…

1. $10 movie ticket, $6 drink, and $6 popcorn _____

2. Two $18 shirts with a buy one, get one half-off sale _____

3. Four coffees at $1.80 each _____

4. $4 fresh pasta, $4 grated Parmesan cheese, $2 parsley, $2.50 lettuce, and $4 tomatoes _____

5. Buy three, get one free on tires that are $70 each, plus a $75 installation fee _____

6. Five-day car rental for $42 each day _____

7. $1.90 per bus ride, three rides needed _____

8. $50 meal split between 4 people _____

9. $180 plane ticket plus $55 in fees _____

10. $72 gift split between 3 people _____

> PROBLEM SOLVING

Practical Math

Use a calculator and pen and paper as needed.

Example: $10 plus 10% simple interest is $11.

CALCULATING TOTALS WITH PERCENTAGES. How much is...

1. $10 plus 8% tax _____

2. $1.00 plus 9% tax _____

3. $30 meal with a 15% tip _____

4. $140,000 loan plus 5% simple interest _____

5. $300,000 loan plus 2.5% simple interest _____

6. $2,400 bill plus 23% simple interest _____

7. $35 plus 8.5% tax _____

8. $70,000 salary plus a 2% raise _____

9. $75,000 salary plus a 3% raise _____

10. $1,200 plus 15% tax _____

> PROBLEM SOLVING

Practical Math

Use a calculator and pen and paper as needed.

CALCULATING TOTALS. How much is…

1. Monthly payment for a $435, 6-month car insurance premium _____

2. Monthly payment for a one-year $1,800 hospital bill _____

3. Daily rate for a one-week $245 car rental _____

4. Yearly payment for a 30-year $300,000 mortgage _____

5. Yearly payment for a 10-year $40,000 loan _____

6. Minute rate for a 20-minute $12 international phone call _____

7. Daily rate for a 2-day $450 hotel stay _____

8. Minute rate for a 30-minute $45 massage _____

9. Monthly payment for a 2-year $20,000 loan _____

10. Daily rate for a 3-week $7,000 cruise _____

PROBLEM SOLVING

Practical Math

Use a calculator and pen and paper as needed.

CALCULATING TIMES. What time is…

1. 30 minutes before 8:00 am _____

2. 4 hours before 11:00 pm _____

3. 14 hours before 2:00 pm _____

4. 3 hours and 30 minutes before 9:30 am_____

5. 7 hours and 45 minutes after 10:45 pm _____

6. 16 hours after 7:00 pm _____

7. 25 minutes before 6:40 am _____

8. 2 hours and 50 minutes before 3:00 pm _____

9. 4 hours and 45 minutes before 12:15 pm _____

10. 8 hours and 10 minutes after 1:55 am _____

> PROBLEM SOLVING

Practical Math

Use a calculator and pen and paper as needed.

CALCULATING TIMES.

1. Your dentist is 15 minutes away. What time should you leave your house to be right on time for an 8:30 am appointment?
   _____

2. The bank is 20 minutes away. What time should you leave your house to arrive when it opens at 10:00 am?
   _____

3. The movie is 2 hours and 15 minutes long. It started at 3:35 pm. What time does it end?
   _____

4. Your doctor appointment is at 2:30 pm. You need to arrive 15 minutes early, and you live 25 minutes away. When should you leave your house?
   _____

5. Your son's airplane lands at 9:45 pm and his luggage arrives 15 minutes later. You live 50 minutes away. What time should you leave your house to arrive right when the luggage does?
   _____

PROBLEM SOLVING

Math in Everyday Life

Practice your math skills with the following tasks:

ROAD TRIPS. Choose a fun road trip destination. Use an atlas or Google Maps.
- Calculate the total distance.
- Plan how many stops you will take.
- Calculate how much you'll spend on gas or tickets.

WEEKLY ADS. Get a copy of the weekly ad from the local grocery store.
- Decide on a budget for a week's worth of groceries.
- Write a list of all the items you need.
- Using the weekly ad, write down the price of all the items you need.
- Calculate how much your total cost would be.

RESTAURANT MENUS. Get a copy of a restaurant's take-out menu.
- Set a budget.
- Write a list of all the items you want.
- Add tax and a tip.
- Calculate how much your total will be.

Medical Team Phone Numbers

PRIMARY CARE PROVIDER _____

PHARMACY _____

HEALTH INSURANCE COMPANY_____

THERAPY COMPANY _____

HOSPITAL _____

WALK-IN CLINIC _____

URGENT CARE _____

EMERGENCY ROOM _____

SPECIALISTS _____

_____

_____

THERAPISTS _____

_____

_____

PROBLEM SOLVING

Emergency Plan

In the event of disasters and emergencies, it is recommended that every household has an Emergency Plan. Visit ready.gov for more information (The Department of Homeland Security, 2021).

EMERGENCY WARNINGS. I will receive emergency warnings via *(e.g. radio)*

_____

SHELTER PLAN. I will seek shelter at *(e.g., home, mass shelter)*

_____

_____

FOOD AND WATER. I will have the following items ready *(e.g. bottled water)*

_____

_____

SUPPLIES. I will have the following supplies ready *(e.g., sleeping bags, matches)*

_____

_____

EVACUATION ROUTE. I will evacuate via *(e.g. south to John's house)*

_____

_____

COMMUNICATION. My household communication plan is *(e.g., out-of-town contact, emergency meeting place)*

_____

_____

PROBLEM SOLVING

Sequencing

Place the steps in the correct order, using the numbers 1 through 4.

☐ Put the pot on the stove.
☐ Wait for the water to boil.
☐ 1 Fill up the pot with water.
☐ Turn on the stove.

☐ Put the bread in the toaster.
☐ Open the bread bag.
☐ Add butter to the toast.
☐ Push the lever down on the toaster.

☐ Write a letter.
☐ Get paper and a pen.
☐ Place envelope in mailbox.
☐ Place letter in envelope.

☐ Pour ingredients into frying pan.
☐ Add cheese to bowl.
☐ Combine all ingredients.
☐ Mix eggs and salt in a large bowl.

☐ Turn the light-switch off.
☐ Place new lightbulb in.
☐ Notice the lightbulb went out.
☐ Remove old lightbulb.

☐ Turn on the tap.
☐ Rinse off soap.
☐ Wash hands.
☐ Add soap.

Sequencing

Place the steps in the correct order, using the numbers 1 through 5.

☐ Receive a diagnosis.

☐ Sign in at the doctor's office.

[1] Make an appointment.

☐ Get your temperature taken.

☐ Drive to the doctor's office.

☐ Pour in clean water.

☐ Wait for coffee to brew.

☐ Add cream and sugar.

☐ Remove old coffee grounds.

☐ Pour a cup of coffee.

☐ Read the menu.

☐ Drive to the restaurant.

☐ Order at the counter.

☐ Eat your meal.

☐ Wait for your meal.

☐ Drain the pasta.

☐ Place cold water in a pot.

☐ Place pasta in boiling water.

☐ Bring the pot of water to a boil.

☐ Eat the pasta.

PROBLEM SOLVING

Sequencing

Place the steps in the correct order, using the numbers 1 through 5.

- [ ] Mother's Day
- [1] New Year's Day
- [ ] Fourth of July

- [ ] Christmas
- [ ] Halloween

- [ ] Monday
- [ ] Wednesday
- [ ] Friday

- [ ] Saturday
- [ ] Tuesday

- [ ] February
- [ ] March
- [ ] October

- [ ] November
- [ ] January

- [ ] Death
- [ ] Adulthood
- [ ] Adolescence

- [ ] Birth
- [ ] Infancy

PROBLEM SOLVING

Sequencing

Place the steps in the correct order, using the numbers 1 through 5.

☐ Mile   [1] Millimeter

☐ Yard   ☐ Foot

☐ Inch

☐ Teaspoon   ☐ Cup

☐ Gallon   ☐ Tablespoon

☐ Pint

☐ Dime   ☐ Nickel

☐ Quarter   ☐ Penny

☐ Half-dollar

☐ Hundred   ☐ Thousand

☐ Negative one   ☐ Zero

☐ Million

PROBLEM SOLVING

Make a Schedule

Use your problem solving skills to fill out a schedule for each scenario below. Not all of the spaces need to filled. Cross out information in the paragraph after you've added it to the schedule.

---

1. Bonnie has a dentist appointment at 11 am. She needs to arrive 30 minutes early to fill out some forms. After her appointment, she's meeting a friend for lunch at 12:30 pm. 1 hour after that, she and her friend will go shopping at the mall (4 events).

10:00 am _____   12:00 pm _____
10:30 am _____   12:30 pm _____
11:00 am _____   1:00 pm _____
11:30 am _____   1:30 pm _____

2. Unja has a flight that leaves at 4 pm. She wants to arrive at the airport 2 hours before her flight. Before she leaves for her trip, she needs to drop off a check at the bank. The flight is 2 hours long. She plans to have dinner with her friends 1 hour after she lands (5 events).

1:00 pm _____   5:00 pm _____
2:00 pm _____   6:00 pm _____
3:00 pm _____   7:00 pm _____
4:00 pm _____   8:00 pm _____

PROBLEM SOLVING

3. Your favorite speech therapist has 4, 1-hour-long therapy appointments this morning. Before that, she will have coffee at her favorite cafe. She's meeting a colleague for lunch at noon. Before heading to a meeting downtown, she will see 1 more patient in the afternoon (8 events).

7:00 am _____   11:00 am _____
8:00 am _____   12:00 pm _____
9:00 am _____   1:00 pm _____
10:00 am _____   2:00 pm _____

4. The country veterinarian allots 1 hour per animal visit. This afternoon, she will treat a horse and a cow. But first, she has a big breakfast with her family and then takes a shower. Her first appointment is in the office at 9 am with a dog. Before a lunch meeting at noon, she sees a cat and then a ferret (8 events).

7:00 am _____   11:00 am _____
8:00 am _____   12:00 pm _____
9:00 am _____   1:00 pm _____
10:00 am _____   2:00 pm _____

5. Before they arrive on Mars, the astronauts need to train, board the spacecraft, and dock at the International Space Station. They will collect rock samples before returning back to Earth (6 events).

First _____   Fourth _____
Second _____   Fifth _____
Third _____   Sixth _____

PROBLEM SOLVING

6. Jude had a date at 7 pm. 1 hour before the date, he caught the train and 45 minutes after that, he bought a bouquet at a floral shop. 10 minutes later, Jude checked his hair and teeth in a mirror. After an hour-and-a-half-long dinner, the couple went to the movie theater. He arrived back home 6 hours after he first left (write in the 6 events and the times that they happened).

_____ _____   _____ _____

_____ _____   _____ _____

_____ _____   _____ _____

7. The cat show begins right at 8 am, although registration opens 1 hour earlier. The contestants have 30 minutes to prepare their cats before the judges arrive on the floor. Judging is scheduled to last 3 hours. The results are finalized 1 hour and 30 minutes after the judges finish. Best Cat awards are presented at 2:00 pm (write in the 6 events and the times that they happened).

_____ _____   _____ _____

_____ _____   _____ _____

_____ _____   _____ _____

8. We arrived in Bali on the 10th, just 2 days after flying into Java. On our last day in Java, we went hiking. We also hiked on our 2nd and 4th days in Bali! The highlight of our trip was a day at Lake Toba in Sumatra on the 15th (write in the 6 events and the dates they happened).

_____ _____   _____ _____

_____ _____   _____ _____

_____ _____   _____ _____

> **PROBLEM SOLVING**

Meal Planning

Consider the following tips to make meal planning easier and your meals healthier. Always adhere to your doctor-recommended diet.

KEEP IT SIMPLE. Delicious, healthy meals can have 5 or fewer ingredients.

KEEP A LIST. Place a whiteboard or magnetic memo pad on your refrigerator and write down your grocery list throughout the week. You can also use a Notes app on your smart phone.

PLAN ONE MEAL AT A TIME. Decide what you want to eat. After planning a meal, add the items you need to your grocery list. Move on to the next meal.

USE FROZEN OR CANNED INGREDIENTS. If preparing fresh fruits and vegetables is too challenging or time-consuming, canned or frozen produce can be a nutritious option. Avoid added sugars and salt.

GROCERY SHOP AT THE SAME TIME EVERY WEEK. Get in a routine to decrease the chance of forgetting to shop and running out of food.

ADD SPICES FOR FLAVOR. Consider spices such as paprika, cumin, and rosemary to add flavor in place of butter and salt.

Meals this Week

	BREAKFAST	LUNCH	DINNER	SNACKS
MONDAY				
TUESDAY				
WEDNESDAY				
THURSDAY				
FRIDAY				
SATURDAY				
SUNDAY				

Groceries for Meals

MEAL	GROCERIES NEEDED

Grocery List

GROCERIES NEEDED			
PRODUCE		CANNED FOOD	
DELI		BOXED FOOD	
MEAT & SEAFOOD		BAKING	
DAIRY		OTHER BREAD	
BAKERY		CEREAL	
FROZEN		CONDIMENTS	
BEVERAGES		SNACKS	
PERSONAL CARE		MISC.	

PROBLEM SOLVING | *Page 1 of 2*

Balance a Checkbook

Add the following transactions into the checkbook on the next page.

---

1. $58 at Home Shop on 12/10.

2. $38 at GoGo Gas Station on 12/10.

3. $560 income check on 12/20.

4. $930 rent check, #305 on 12/27.

5. $90 utility check, #306 on 12/27.

6. $5.15 at Caffeine Cup on 12/29.

7. $13.55 at Big Guy's Burgers on 12/30.

PROBLEM SOLVING

Page 2 of 2

Check #	Date	Description	Payment, withdrawal	Fee	Deposit, credit	Total
	12/05	Direct Deposit			$800.00	$910.00

PROBLEM SOLVING *Page 1 of 2*

Balance a Checkbook

Add the following transactions into the checkbook on the next page.

---

1. $5.50 at Philly's Coffee on 05/04.

2. $18.50 at Salon Salon on 05/04.

3. $185 for utilities on 05/07.

4. $998 deposit on 05/10.

5. $20 donation to Scout Troop, check #225, on 05/11.

6. $50 deposit on 05/18.

7. $145 at Herb's Herbary, check #226, on 05/19.

8. $3.50 at Caffeine Cup on 05/19.

9. $998 deposit on 05/25.

PROBLEM SOLVING

Page 2 of 2

Check #	Date	Description	Payment, withdrawal	Fee	Deposit, credit	Total
	05/03	Golden Dragon Cafe	$25.75			$389

PROBLEM SOLVING *Page 1 of 2*

Balance a Checkbook

Add the following transactions into the checkbook on the next page.

---

1. $25 for Connie's Birthday, check #491, on 10/02.

2. $25 for June's Birthday, check #492, on 10/03.

3. $35.10 at Dairy on the Double on 10/03.

4. $775 deposit on 10/10.

5. $32.90 at Stone Cinemas on 10/11.

6. $31.00 at Rosco's Bar on 10/11.

7. $78.20 at Ergomart on 10/12.

8. $11.45 at Pizza Pie on 10/12.

9. $7.40 at Starbucks on 10/12.

10. $400.95 at Ridge Lodge, check #493, on 10/25.

PROBLEM SOLVING

Page 2 of 2

Check #	Date	Description	Payment, withdrawal	Fee	Deposit, credit	Total
490	10/02	Brianna's birthday	$25.00			$550.10

PROBLEM SOLVING — Page 1 of 2

Everyday Math

Review the menu on the next page then answer the questions.

WHAT IS THE TOTAL COST OF...

1. Coffee and biscotti?

   _____

2. Hot chocolate and slice of cake?

   _____

3. Mocha, muffin, and scone?

   _____

4. Tea plus a 20% tip?

   _____

5. Bagel and fruit cup plus a $2 tip?

   _____

PROBLEM SOLVING

Reya's Café

DRINKS
- Coffee $2.50
- Tea $2.00
- Latte $4.00
- Cappuccino $4.00
- Mocha $4.50
- Hot Chocolate $3.50

SNACKS
- Biscotti $2.50
- Bagel $3.50
- Muffin $3.00
- Scone $3.50
- Cake Slice $4.50
- Fruit Cup $4.00

> **PROBLEM SOLVING** — *Page 1 of 2*

Everyday Math

Review the menu on the next page then answer the questions.

WHAT IS THE TOTAL COST OF...

1. Burger and fries?
   _____

2. Cheeseburger with bacon?
   _____

3. Fries with gravy and cheese curds?
   _____

4. Bacon burger with fries and a drink?
   _____

5. Burger with special sauce and fries with special sauce?
   _____

PROBLEM SOLVING

KAZU'S BURGERS

BURGER $6.00
+ CHEDDAR CHEESE $1.00
+BACON $2.00
+ SPECIAL SAUCE $1.00

FRIES $5.00
+ SPECIAL SAUCE $1.00
+ GRAVY AND CHEESE CURDS $4.00

DRINKS $2.50

PROBLEM SOLVING

Page 1 of 2

Everyday Math

Review the menu on the next page then answer the questions.

WHAT IS THE TOTAL COST OF...

1. Cheddar cheese and multigrain crackers?

2. Brie, hard salami, and dark chocolate?

3. Gorgonzola, gouda, and licorice?

4. Rosemary crackers, cheese crackers, blackberry preserves, and apple butter?

5. Muenster cheese, prosciutto, rosemary crackers, and hard candy?

PROBLEM SOLVING

Fifty Shades of Gruyere
Seattle's Finest Cheese Shop

CHEESE, $5 ea
 Aged Cheddar, Brie, Muenster, Gorgonzola, Gouda

CRACKERS, $3 ea
 Multigrain, Cracked Pepper, Rosemary, Cheese

MEAT, $6 ea
 Summer Sausage, Prosciutto, Hard Salami, Turkey Sausage

SPREADS, $2.50 ea
 Orange Marmalade, Blackberry Preserves, Apple Butter

SWEETS, $3 ea
 Hard Candy, Dark Chocolate, Peppermint, Licorice

PROBLEM SOLVING

Everyday Math

Review the menu on the next page then answer the questions.

WHAT IS THE TOTAL COST OF...

1. Cheese burger and fries?

2. House salad and chicken noddle soup?

3. Grilled cheese sandwich and tomato soup?

4. Bacon burger, BLT, turkey club, and two drinks?

5. Two chicken burgers and two drinks plus a 20% tip?

6. Choose one side, one burger, and one drink. What is the total cost?

PROBLEM SOLVING

Wagoneer Diner

SIDES
House Salad $5.00
Caesar Salad $4.50
Fries $4.00
House fries, waffle fries, or sweet potato fries

BURGERS
House Hamburger $9.00
1/3 pound patty, mayo, lettuce, tomato, and pickles
Cheese Burger $10.50
1/3 pound patty, mayo, lettuce, tomato, pickles and your choice of cheddar, pepper jack, or American cheese
Bacon Burger $12.00
1/3 pound patty, mayo, lettuce, tomato, pickles, your choice of cheese, and 4 slices of thick-cut bacon
Chicken Burger $10.00
Grilled chicken breast, mayo, lettuce, tomato, and grilled onions

SANDWICHES
BLT $8.50
Bacon, lettuce, tomato, cheddar cheese, and mayo
Grilled Cheese $8.00
Your choice of cheddar, pepper jack, or American cheese
Turkey Club $9.00
Oven-roasted chicken breast, honey ham, lettuce, tomato, your choice of cheese, and mayo

SOUP
Tomato $4.00
French Onion $3.50
Broccoli Cheddar $4.50
Chicken Noddle $4.50

DRINKS
Soda, milk, coffee, tea, juice $2.00
Free refills

PROBLEM SOLVING | *Page 1 of 2*

Everyday Math

Review the receipt on the next page then answer the questions. Use a calculator and pen and paper as needed.

---

1. How much is each mango?
   _____

2. How much is each avocado?
   _____

3. How much are apples per pound?
   _____

4. How much is whipped topping?
   _____

5. What is your grand total?
   _____

PROBLEM SOLVING

Page 2 of 2

Shoppalot Market

===========================

4	Mango	$10.76
2	Avocado	$5.98
	Apple (*2.5 lbs*)	$3.75
6	Banana	$3.54
1	Whipped Topping	$X.XX
1	Ginger Ale Soda	$1.89

===========================

SUBTOTAL	$29.91
SALES TAX	$02.39
GRAND TOTAL	**$XX.XX**

CREDIT SALE
ACCT #: ************VISA 0411
08/10/2023   06:15 PM
TRANS #: 00193847219

PROBLEM SOLVING

Everyday Math

Review the receipt on the next page then answer the questions. Use a calculator and pen and paper as needed.

---

1. How much are hot dogs and buns total?
   _____

2. How much are ketchup and mustard?
   _____

3. What percent is the liquor tax (to the nearest percent)?
   _____

4. How much is beer plus tax?
   _____

5. What is your grand total?
   _____

PROBLEM SOLVING

Page 2 of 2

```
       Thank you for shopping at
              Big Box Store

           9055 Sebastian Lane
           Awnpoint, IN 46460

02/14/2022                        08:45 AM
Term ID: ****004
Cashier: Andrew

Item Count: 8
==========================================
1 BOTTLED WATER 24 CT            $5.99
1 BUNS HOT DOG 8 CT              $3.69
1 ALL BEEF HOT DOG               $5.99
1 SAUERKRAUT 16 OZ               $3.99
1 KETCHUP 12 OZ                  $2.19
1 MUSTARD 8 OZ                   $1.89
1 MARSHMALLOW LRG 11.5 OZ        $2.39
1 BEER 6 CT                      $6.99
==========================================
SUBTOTAL                         $33.12
SALES TAX                        $0.00
LIQUOR TAX                       $0.69
GRAND TOTAL                      $XX.XX

CREDIT SALE
ACCT #: ************VISA 0411
REF #: 245891
AUTH CODE: 182223
```

| PROBLEM SOLVING | *Page 1 of 2*

Everyday Math

Review the nutrition label on the next page then answer the questions. Use a calculator and pen and paper as needed.

---

1. How many calories are in two servings?
   _____

2. How many grams of fat are in one serving?
   _____

3. What percent daily value of sodium are there in two servings?
   _____

4. How many grams of fiber are there in half of one serving?
   _____

5. How many calories are there in the entire container?
   _____

PROBLEM SOLVING

Page 2 of 2

Stars & Stripes RANCH DRESSING

Nutrition Facts

64 servings per container

Serving size   **2 tablespoons**

Amount per serving

Calories   **545**

	% Daily Value*
Total Fat 8g	10%
Saturated Fat 2g	7%
Trans Fat 0g	
Cholesterol <5mg	1%
Sodium 250mg	11%
Total Carbohydrate 17g	7%
Dietary Fiber 1g	4%
Total Sugars 1g	
Includes 0g Added Sugars	0%
Protein 5g	8%

Not a significant source of vitamin D, calcium, iron, and potassium.

*The % Daily Value (DV) tells you how much a nutrient in a serving of food contributes to a daily diet. 2,000 calories a day is used for general nutrition advice.

PROBLEM SOLVING

Everyday Math

Review the advertisement on the next page then answer the questions.

WHAT IS THE TOTAL COST OF...

1. 2 pounds of sirloin steak?

   _____

2. 3 pounds of bacon?

   _____

3. 2 pounds of bacon and butter?

   _____

4. A pound-and-a-half of salmon and 3 lemons?

   _____

5. 6 kabobs, salt, and pepper?

   _____

Problem Solving

Page 2 of 2

Grocery Mart
Weekly Deals

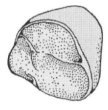
Ham $5.99 lb

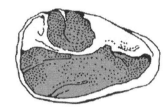
Sirloin Steaks $7.99 lb

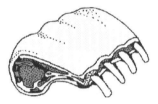
Pork Ribs $4.99 lb

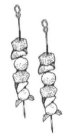
Pork Kabobs $4 ea

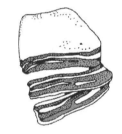
Farm Cut Bacon $2.99 lb

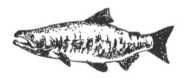
Atlantic Salmon $9.99 lb

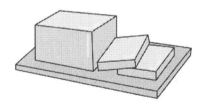
Local Butter $4.39

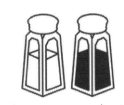
Salt or Pepper $1.29

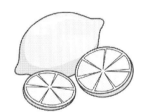
Large Lemons $0.69

PROBLEM SOLVING *Page 1 of 2*

Everyday Math

Review the bank statement on the next page then answers the questions.

---

1. What is the balance after the deposit on 04/01/2022?
   _____

2. How much was spent at SaveDollars.com?
   _____

3. How much was spent at Gas N Go?
   _____

4. What is the balance after the deposit on 04/15/2022?
   _____

5. What was the beginning balance?
   _____

Hoedown Credit Union

Statement Ending 04/30/2022

RETURN SERVICE REQUESTED

Zeke Greenup
732 Greenup Lane
Horsetail, MT 59090

HYRULE CREDIT UNION CHECKING-XX0498

Primary Checking

Account Summary

Date	Description	Amount
04/01/2022	Beginning Balance	$XXX.XX
	3 Credits This Period	$3,300.50
	20 Debits This Period	
04/30/2022	Ending Balance	$1,611.04

Account Activity

Post Date	Description	Debits	Credits	Balance
04/01/2022	Check #119	$800.00		$187.56
04/01/2022	DIRECT DEP		$1,600.00	$XXXX.XX
04/04/2022	Greenup Diner	$37.67		$1749.89
04/04/2022	Sweet Treats	$14.99		$1734.90
04/06/2022	City of Hoedown	$234.00		$1500.90
04/08/2022	SaveDollars.com	$XX.XX		$1411.36
04/09/2022	ATM DEPOSIT		$100.00	$1511.36
04/12/2022	Gas N Go	$XX.XX		$1476.13
04/12/2022	Gussy Burger	$17.14		$1458.99
04/15/2022	DIRECT DEP		$1600.50	$XXXX.XX
04/16/2022	Saddle Mart	$886.86		$2172.63

VISUAL NEGLECT

Visual neglect is a visual perceptual disorder that results in inattention to one side of the visual field. The goal of treatment is to increase awareness of the affected side. Choose visual neglect goals and techniques based on the patient's previous and current levels of functioning, amount of support available, motivation, insight into deficits, and other relevant factors.

Visual neglect treatment includes:
- Visual scanning, anchors, guides, and imagery and compensatory techniques
- Environmental modifications

Some patients may also benefit from prism adaptation, eye-patching, or mental imagery techniques. See asha.org for more information.

Limb activation and constraint-induced movement therapy can also improve outcomes. Refer to occupational or physical therapy.

VISUAL NEGLECT

Therapist Instructions

EVALUATIONS.
- Cognitive screens with a visuospatial section include the *MoCA*, *MMSE*, and *SLUMS*.
- The *Catherine Bergego Scale* (Chen et al., 2012) is a functional scale found to effectively detect mild neglect (Grattan & Woodbury, 2017).
- Formal cognitive batteries include the *Test of Everyday Attention* and parts of the *D-KEFS* and *WAIS-IV*.
- Informal evaluations often include tasks such as cancellation, reading aloud, scanning a picture, reading clocks, and copying written information.

DAY ONE OF TREATMENT. Provide the following handouts, as needed:
- Homework Log, Monthly Calendar, Visuospatial Impairments, Environmental Modifications, Lighthouse Technique, Reading Strategies
- Highlight key points on the handouts, then review with your patients. Ask questions to make sure they understand the content. Answer any questions they may have.

FOR THERAPIST EYES ONLY. Therapist treatment guides are marked with a gray background. Some caregivers and patients may benefit from having a copy.
- Practical Tasks and Simple Tasks

ANOSOGNOSIA. Visual neglect treatment is often complicated by patients' reduced awareness of their deficit. Treat anosognosia using the 'M' of TEACH-M (page 184) and other strategies to improve self-awareness (Blake et al., 2016).

STRATEGIES. Choose 2-3 of the most useful strategies and focus on those with your patient.
- Review the selected strategies, provide a model, then ask for return demonstrations.
- Lighthouse Technique, Reading Strategies, Organized Scanning

VISUAL NEGLECT

Page 2 of 2

ENVIRONMENTAL MODIFICATIONS (PAGE 254). Review this worksheet with the caregiver so they can help make the modifications.

SIMPLE TASKS. Simple tasks, like letter cancellation, can be a good way to practice visual scanning strategies and to increase patient confidence. However, these skills tend not to generalize to real life. Quickly transition to more practical tasks, such as reading short words.

MAZES (PAGE 265). Make this task measurable by timing how long it takes to complete the maze and/or by measuring cues.

WORD SEARCH PUZZLES (PAGE 268). Make this task measurable by creating a time limit or timing how long it takes to complete the puzzle and/or by measuring cues.

ONE-SIDED PRINTING (PAGES 272–275, 290–293). Some tasks include two pages: one with reading material/maps and the other with questions. Print these one-sided (so the patient doesn't need to flip the paper back and forth).

QUESTIONNAIRE (PAGE 276) & APPLICATION (PAGE 278). Cue patients to use their scanning strategies.

READING MATERIAL. See the Memory and Aphasia chapters for more reading material.

REFERRING TO A VISION SPECIALIST. If you suspect visual field cuts or more complex visual processing deficits, consider a referral to an occupational therapist or physician who specializes in this area.

VISUAL NEGLECT

Contents

Practical Tasks...................................	251
Simple Tasks......................................	252
Visuospatial Impairments.....................	253
Environmental Modifications.................	254
Lighthouse Technique..........................	255
Reading Strategies..............................	256
Cancellation Task................................	258
Connect-the-Dots................................	260
Mazes..	265
Organized Scanning............................	267
Word Search Puzzles............................	268
Everyday Reading...............................	272
Health Inventory *(Questionnaire)*.............	276
Application..	278
Reading Material................................	280
Reading Maps....................................	285

SEE ALSO

Reading a Calendar.......................	122
Write in Appointments...................	126
Remembering Reading Material......	165
Everyday Math.............................	228
Paragraphs..................................	389
Reading......................................	395
Everyday Reading.........................	399

VISUAL NEGLECT

Practical Tasks

WRITING. Refer to the Aphasia chapter (page 330) for writing tasks.

READ MAPS. Find a map (such as a mall directory or hospital map) and have your patient locate different points using finger scanning. Have them trace the most direct route between two points.
- The patient can also draw a map of their current location (e.g., home, skilled nursing facility).

DESCRIBE VISUAL SCENES. Present the photos on pages 428 and have your patient describe them in as much detail as possible.

READ WEEKLY ADS. Have your patient find certain items in the ad using take it slow, anchors, and/or finger scanning.

READ MAGAZINES AND BOOKS. Have your patient read aloud while using finger scanning, underlining, and/or organized scanning.

FILL OUT APPLICATIONS AND SURVEYS. Hospitals typically mail surveys after a visit. Have your patient use take it slow, anchors, finger scanning, underlining, and/or organized scanning to complete this task.

VISUAL NEGLECT

Simple Tasks

Start with these simpler visual neglect tasks to practice scanning strategies and to increase confidence.

CANCELLATION TASK (PAGE 258). Have your patient cross out specific items in a series of letters, numbers, or symbols.

CONNECT-THE-DOTS (PAGE 260). Have your patient use organized scanning (page 267) and "take it slow" during this task.

MAZES (PAGE 265). Have your patient use finger scanning and "take it slow."

WORD SEARCH PUZZLES (PAGE 268). Have your patient use finger scanning, anchors, and organized scanning to complete this task.

CARD GAMES. Have your patient use the lighthouse technique to play games such as Solitaire, Go Fish, or War.

"I SPY™" AND "WHERE'S WALDO®" BOOKS. Have your patient use organized scanning, "take it slow," and the lighthouse technique (page 255).

VISUAL NEGLECT

Visuospatial Impairments

Common visuospatial impairments include:

VISUAL NEGLECT. A disorder that causes inattention to one side of the visual field (either left or right side, although most commonly left). It is caused by damage to the brain *(Sutton, 2014)*. Although the person can 'see', their brain fails to pay attention to that side. Therapy can help increase visual attention.

VISUAL FIELD CUTS. A vision disorder that causes "true" blindness (when the brain doesn't process visual information) to part of the visual field *(Barclay, 2020)*. It is caused by damage to the brain. Talk to your therapist and doctor if a visual field cut is suspected. There are specialists who can help.

VISUAL NEGLECT

Environmental Modifications

WALLS AND DOORWAYS. Place brightly colored tape (masking tape or painter's tape) on the edges of doorways, walls, and tables.

COMPUTER. Stick bright post-it notes on the affected side of the computer screen.

REARRANGE FURNITURE. Reduce the risk of the patient running into objects or tripping. Create straight walking paths and as much open space as possible in rooms the patient spends time in. Remove unneeded furniture.

USING THEIR "GOOD" SIDE. Sit on the patient's un-affected side while you speak with them so that they pay attention to you.

CLEAR CLUTTER. Declutter floors and tabletops. If an item hasn't been used in the past year, get rid of it. Take away at least some knick-knacks that are at eye-level or table-level—these tend to be especially distracting.

ORGANIZE. Organize items by placing them in separate bins. Label the bins. Keep items in the same place so that they're easier to find.
- *For example, you may have separate bins for spices, beauty products, socks, first aid, etc.*

VISUAL NEGLECT

Lighthouse Technique

Use this technique when reading or when navigating in your environment (Niemeier, 1998), such as when you walk into a different room. Use your hand as a guide by sweeping your hand from left to right as you use this technique.

---

1. Start at the far left, turning your head all the way to the left.
2. Slowly scan from left to right.
3. Turn back to the left and scan from left to right again.

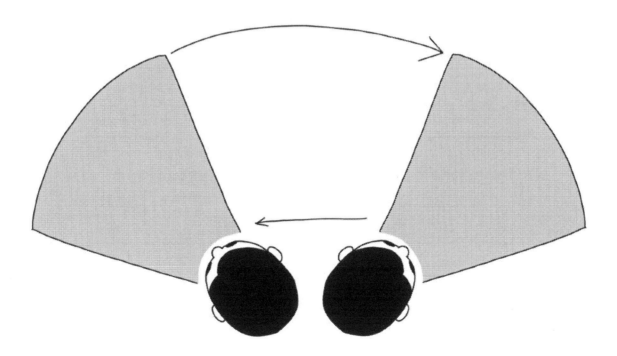

VISUAL NEGLECT *Page 1 of 2*

Reading Strategies

FINGER SCANNING. Use your finger to scan the text as you read from left to right.

MENTAL IMAGERY. Visualize the space of your visual deficit (e.g. left space), close your eyes, and think about what you should be seeing *(Smania et al., 1997)*.

ANCHORS. Place a bright red piece of paper or draw a bold red line down the side of the paper (on the affected side). The color red has been shown to increase attention *(Mehta & Zhu, 2009)*.

PAPER GUIDES. Use a brightly colored strip of paper or blank piece of paper and place it directly underneath the line of text you're reading to help you keep your place.

READ ALOUD. Reading aloud helps you notice if you accidentally skip words or a line of text. Your ears pick up when a sentence doesn't make sense.

VISUAL NEGLECT

UNDERLINE OR HIGHLIGHT. If you are reading something you own (not a library book!), then underline what you're reading with a pencil as you go along. You can also highlight the text as you read.

LARGER TEXT. It's often easier to read larger text. Most library systems have a "Large Print" section and many popular magazines also have a larger text version. If you're reading something on your phone, computer, or tablet, increase the text size in the settings.

TAKE IT SLOW. Pace yourself and remember to give your healing brain extra time to process information. Slow and steady wins this race.

VISUAL NEGLECT

Cancellation Task

Cross out, circle, or mark the letter or symbol indicated. Find all of one letter/symbol first, then move on to the next letter/symbol.

CROSS OUT ALL OF THE "T"s AND "R"s.

V	F	T	E	R	G	C	B	T	R	F	E	D
T	V	D	F	R	T	V	F	R	T	C	D	G
G	F	C	R	T	F	V	G	F	R	C	D	S
R	T	R	T	G	V	T	V	F	D	R	G	E

CROSS OUT ALL OF THE "F"s AND "W"s.

R	F	D	S	X	W	D	R	F	S	W	Q	X
C	F	E	W	W	F	X	D	S	E	Z	A	E
Q	E	T	R	D	W	S	C	D	S	X	Z	D
E	R	Q	S	F	C	D	F	W	S	F	W	F

VISUAL NEGLECT

CROSS OUT ALL OF THE "4"s AND "9"s.

5	3	1	4	9	6	9	4	2	5	7	5	3
4	9	7	6	4	4	9	8	6	4	0	7	4
4	7	8	6	5	4	9	9	7	6	0	7	5
9	8	6	4	3	6	8	6	5	4	7	0	5

CROSS OUT ALL OF THE "%"s AND "$"s.

!	&	#	@	$	#	%	%	#	$	%	@	!
%	$	%	$	@	!	$	#	!	#	$	%	%
%	#	@	!	$	#	@	%	%	$	@	$	$
@	!	#	$	#	%	$	$	@	!	@	%	$

VISUAL NEGLECT

Connect-the-Dots

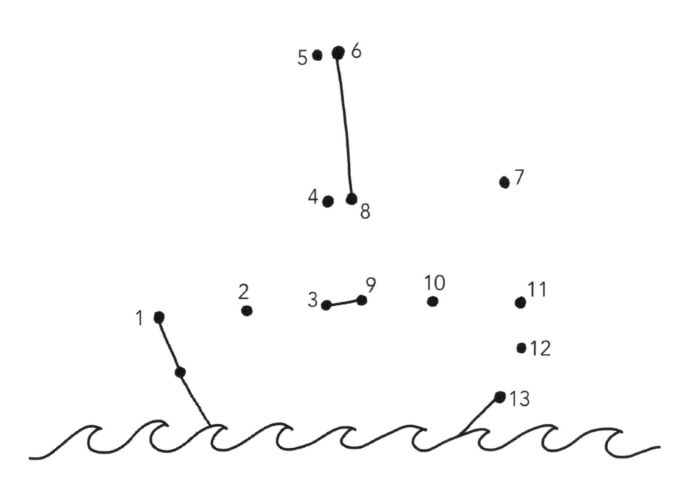

VISUAL NEGLECT

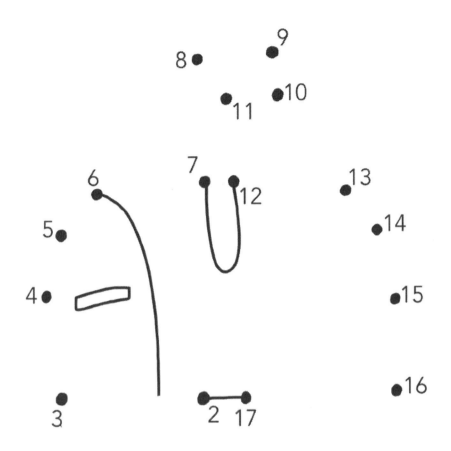

VISUAL NEGLECT

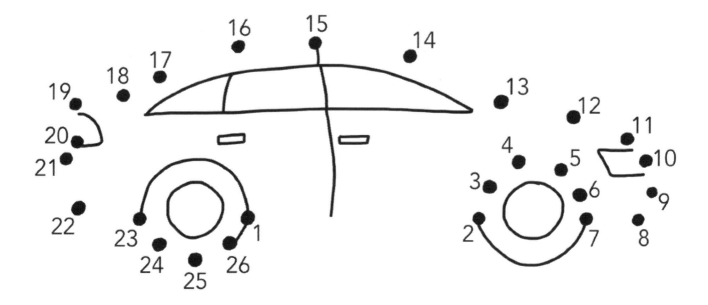

VISUAL NEGLECT

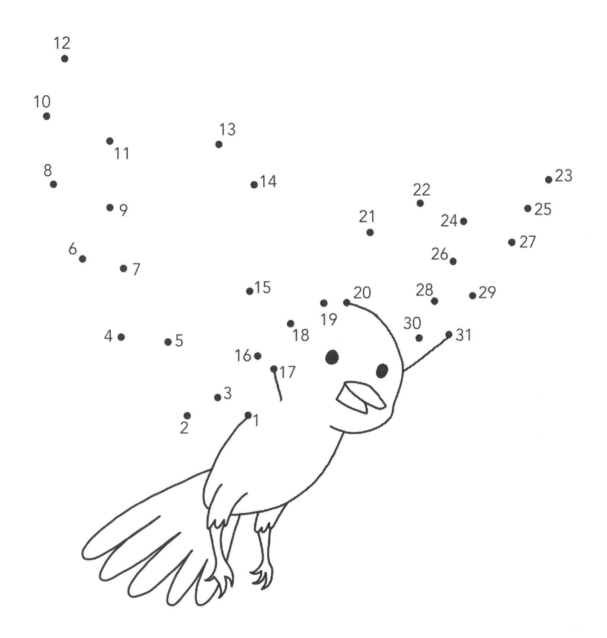

VISUAL NEGLECT

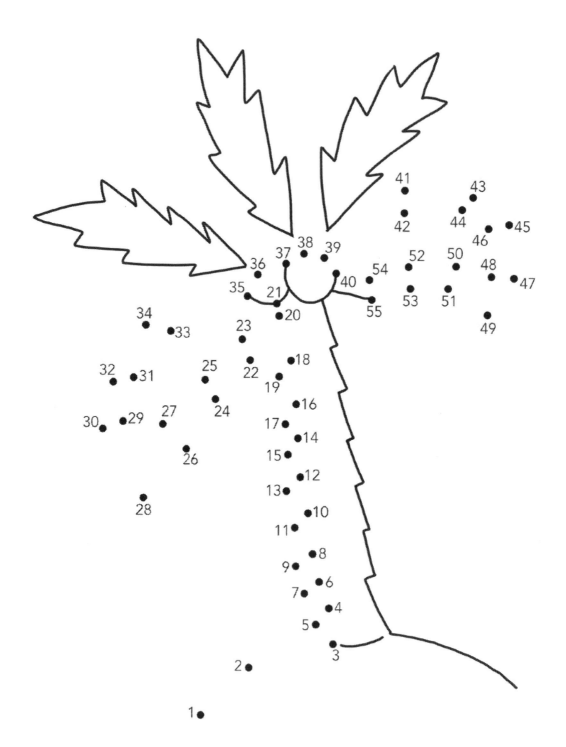

VISUAL NEGLECT

Mazes

Use your scanning techniques to solve the following mazes.

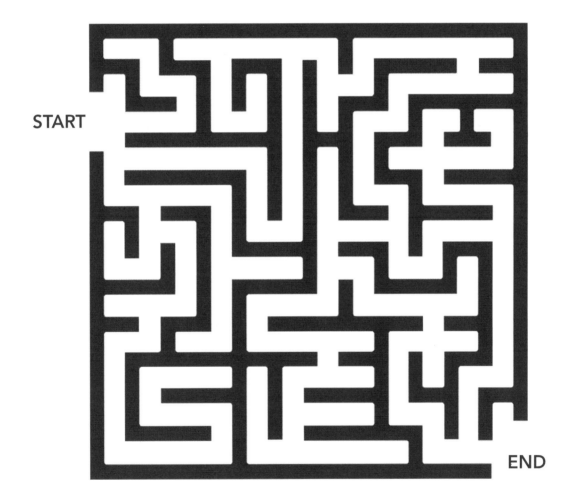

VISUAL NEGLECT

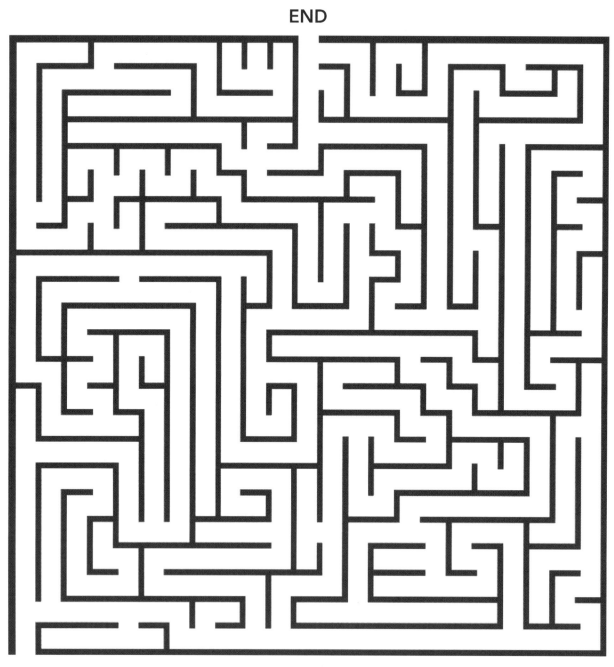

| VISUAL NEGLECT |

Organized Scanning

Use these tips to look for specific information while you're reading (e.g. phone number on a credit card statement). They can also help you complete word search puzzles.

---

1. Start at the **top left** corner of the page.
2. Use your finger to scan **left to right**, looking for the **first letter** of the first word.
    - *For example, when looking for the telephone number on a credit card statement, search for the letter "T."*
3. Once you get to the end of the sentence, go back to the left and scan the next sentence.
4. Continue until you find the word; mark the word by highlighting or circling it.
5. Move to the next word and repeat steps 1-5.

If you have a hard time finding a word, move on to the next word, and come back to it later.

B	K	G	B	V	O
A	M	E	F	Y	R
N	V	F	Z	C	A
A	P	P	L	E	N
N	L	I	M	E	G
A	M	O	B	A	E

ORANGE   APPLE

LIME   BANANA

```
S T O J M Y P
T P G L A J A
A E S T R D P
P N Y A K T E
L C H P E P R
E I B E R G A
R L E I A N M
```

PAPER   PENCIL   STAPLER
TAPE   MARKER

```
F W S G G A O V C J
P N H Y J T E C S J
A R O W V I O G H F
O D C P L A V L E G
D I R T N C E L A L
T W S H O V E L R O
F L O W E R S C S V
P L A N T E R S K E
P L O W P I R Y M S
C W E H W K M H U K
```

SHOVEL   SHEARS   DIRT

GLOVES   PLANTERS   FLOWERS

PLOW

Words may appear backwards, upside down, or diagonal.

```
A X C D R C O G K M V M E D Q Q
S N N O T G N I H S A W D N O A
S W U T Y C D O D A T K B Y C D
O Z N H P I I S R N V C P N I A
R Z E X U K W A H E M N T C X V
N O A A R I Z O N A G T Y A E E
G D Y S D D E Y M U G O C L M N
G Q U W K W P O P W K A N I W T
A F E O W I N D D Q Z F I F E P
R R T Y D E C A T R Y A M O N Z
S F A A V F Z R R O A U O R V D
H E H A Q R L O V P D D N N N A
A O D N E W X L M L J K T I Q W
T A Z D R G L O U K X I A A H I
U R Y X R F E C T L Y X N G E M
V A P M E E C C G Y R M A G D W
```

WASHINGTON   OREGON   CALIFORNIA
UTAH   IDAHO   NEVADA
NEW MEXICO   COLORADO   ARIZONA
MONTANA

Everyday Reading

Using your reading strategies, read the material on the next page aloud. Then answer the questions below.

---

1. What is the name of this recipe?

2. What is the first ingredient?

3. What is the last ingredient?

4. What is the first step?

5. What number step includes heating up a pan?

VISUAL NEGLECT

Page 2 of 2

Fluffy French Toast

INGREDIENTS
¼ cup flour
1 cup milk
1 pinch salt
3 eggs
½ teaspoon ground cinnamon
1 teaspoon vanilla extract
1 tablespoon white sugar
12 thick slices bread

DIRECTIONS
1. Measure flour into a large mixing bowl. Slowly whisk in the milk.
2. Whisk in the salt, eggs, cinnamon, vanilla extract, and sugar until smooth.
3. Heat a lightly oiled frying pan over medium heat.
4. Soak bread slices, one at a time, until saturated with the egg mixture.
5. Fry bread on each side until golden brown.

VISUAL NEGLECT *Page 1 of 2*

Everyday Reading

Using your reading strategies, read the material on the next page aloud. Then answer the questions below.

---

1. When was this letter written?
   _____

2. Who sent this letter?
   _____

3. Who is this letter for?
   _____

4. How much is due?
   _____

5. When was the Post-op visit?
   _____

VISUAL NEGLECT

Page 2 of 2

COUNTRY HOSPITAL
9595 Fondue Lane
Cheesetown, USA 99999
(800) 555-8080

Dolly Johnson
320 Dairy Lane
Cheesetown, USA 99999

Patient Statement
June 12, 2022

AMOUNT DUE	AMOUNT PAID
$29.00	
Payment Type	
Check	
Discover	American Express
Visa	Mastercard

Account # _____

Expiration Date _____ / _____ / _____

Signature _____

Date _____ / _____ / _____

DATE	DESCRIPTION	FEE	INSURANCE	PATIENT
5/23/22	Post-op visit	$145.00	$116.00	$29.00

Deposit	0-30	31-60	60-90	91-120	Total Bal.	Ins. Bal	Pat. Bal
$0.00	$29	$0.00	$0.00	$0.00	$29.00	$0.00	$29.00

| VISUAL NEGLECT | Page 1 of 2 |

Health Inventory

Using your reading strategies, read the Health Inventory aloud and answer the questions. You can say or write the answers. Feel free to make up any answers.

How true or false are each of the following statements?	Definitely true	Mostly true	Don't know	Mostly false	Definitely false
a. I seem to get sick easier than most people					
b. I am as healthy as anybody I know					
c. I expect my health to get worse					
d. My health is excellent					

During the last 4 weeks, how much have you been bothered by any of the following problems?	Not bothered	Bothered a little	Bothered a lot
a. Stomach pain			
b. Back pain			
c. Pain in your arms, legs, or joints			
d. Headaches			
e. Chest pain			
f. Dizziness			
g. Shortness of breath			
h. Constipation, loose bowels, or diarrhea			

During the last 14 days, how much have you been bothered by any of the following problems?	Not bothered	Bothered a little	Bothered a lot
a. Little interest or pleasure in doing things			
b. Feeling down, depressed, or hopeless			
c. Poor appetite or overeating			
d. Trouble concentrating on activities, such as reading the newspaper or watching television			

Does your health limit you in the following activities?	Yes, limited a lot	Yes, limited a little	No, not limited at all
a. Vigorous activities, like running			
b. Moderate activities, like pushing a vacuum or playing golf			
c. Lifting or carrying groceries			
d. Climbing several flights of stairs			
e. Bending, kneeling, or stooping			
f. Walking several blocks			
g. Walking one block			
h. Bathing or dressing yourself			

Do you have a family member with a history of any of the following? Please include relation.	
a. Diabetes	
b. High Cholesterol	
c. Heart trouble	
d. High Blood Pressure	
e. Cancer	
f. Glaucoma	
g. Stroke (cerebral vascular accident)	

VISUAL NEGLECT *Page 1 of 2*

Application

Using your reading strategies, read the Application aloud and answer the questions. You can write or say the answers. Feel free to make up any answers.

Basic Information	
Name	Birthdate
Address	Telephone
	Marital Status

Household Members. List all people living in the household.		
Name	Relationship	Birthdate

Favorites	
Hobbies	
Favorite food	
Favorite season	
Favorite holiday	
Favorite music	
Favorite quote	

Family & Friends	
Parents' names	
Immediate family's name(s)	
Best friend's name(s)	
Pet's name(s)	

Values	
What is your definition of success?	
What makes you feel most at peace?	
What is your proudest accomplishment?	
Who in your life are you most proud of?	

Dreams	
What are the top 3 items on your Bucket List?	
A genie grants you 3 wishes. What are they?	
You have the choice to be immortal. Do you choose it? Why or why not?	
What is your number 1 personal goal?	

VISUAL NEGLECT

Reading Material

As you read aloud, use your reading strategies (including finger scanning and placing a red anchor line on the side of the page).

Adventures of Huckleberry Finn
by Mark Twain

You don't know about me, without you have read a book by the name of The Adventures of Tom Sawyer; but that ain't no matter. That book was made by Mr. Mark Twain, and he told the truth, mainly. There was things which he stretched, but mainly he told the truth. That is nothing. I never seen anybody but lied one time or another, without it was Aunt Polly, or the widow, or maybe Mary. Aunt Polly—Tom's Aunt Polly, she is—and Mary, and the Widow Douglas is all told about in that book, which is mostly a true book, with some stretchers, as I said before.

Now the way that the book winds up is this: Tom and me found the money that the robbers hid in the cave, and it made us rich. We got six thousand dollars apiece—all gold. It was an awful sight of money when it was piled up. Well, Judge Thatcher he took it and put it out at interest, and it fetched us a dollar a day apiece all the year round—more than a body could tell what to do with. The Widow Douglas she took me for her son, and allowed she would sivilize me; but it was rough living in the house all the time, considering how dismal regular and decent the widow was in all her ways; and so when I couldn't stand it no longer I lit out. I got into my old rags and my sugar-hogshead again, and was free and satisfied. But Tom Sawyer he hunted me up and said he was going to start a band of robbers, and I might join if I would go back to the widow and be respectable. So I went back.

The widow she cried over me, and called me a poor lost lamb, and she called me a lot of other names, too, but she never meant no harm by it. She put me in them new clothes again, and I couldn't do nothing but sweat and sweat, and feel all cramped up. Well, then, the old thing commenced again. The widow rung a bell for supper, and you had to come to time. When you got to the table you couldn't go right to eating, but you had to wait for the widow to tuck down her head and grumble a little over the victuals, though there warn't really anything the matter with them,—that is, nothing only everything was cooked by itself. In a barrel of odds and ends it is different; things get mixed up, and the juice kind of swaps around, and the things go better.

After supper she got out her book and learned me about Moses and the Bulrushers, and I was in a sweat to find out all about him; but by and by she let it out that Moses had been dead a considerable long time; so then I didn't care no more about him, because I don't take no stock in dead people.

Pretty soon I wanted to smoke, and asked the widow to let me. But she wouldn't. She said it was a mean practice and wasn't clean, and I must try to not do it any more. That is just the way with some people. They get down on a thing when they don't know nothing about it. Here she was a-bothering about Moses, which was no kin to her, and no use to anybody, being gone, you see, yet finding a power of fault with me for doing a thing that had some good in it. And she took snuff, too; of course that was all right, because she done it herself.

Her sister, Miss Watson, a tolerable slim old maid, with goggles on, had just come to live with her, and took a set at me now with a spelling-book. She worked me middling hard for about an hour, and then the widow made her ease up. I couldn't stood it much longer. Then for an hour it was deadly dull, and I was fidgety. Miss Watson would say, "Don't put your feet up there, Huckleberry;" and "Don't scrunch up like that, Huckleberry—set up straight;" and pretty soon she would say, "Don't gap and stretch like that, Huckleberry—why don't you try to behave?" Then she told me all about the bad place, and I said I wished I was there. She got mad then, but I didn't mean no harm. All I wanted was to go somewheres; all I wanted was a change, I warn't particular. She said it was wicked to say what I said; said she wouldn't say it for the whole world; she was going to live so as to go to the good place. Well, I couldn't see no advantage in going where she was going, so I made up my mind I wouldn't try for it. But I never said so, because it would only make trouble, and wouldn't do no good.

Now she had got a start, and she went on and told me all about the good place. She said all a body would have to do there was to go around all day long with a harp and sing, forever and ever. So I didn't think much of it. But I never said so. I asked her if she reckoned Tom Sawyer would go there, and she said not by a considerable sight. I was glad about that, because I wanted him and me to be together. Miss Watson she kept pecking at me, and it got tiresome and lonesome. By and by they fetched the [men] in and had prayers, and then everybody was off to bed. I went up to my room with a piece of candle, and put it on the table. Then I set down in a chair by the window and tried to think of something cheerful, but it warn't no use. I felt so lonesome I most wished I was dead. The stars were shining, and the leaves rustled in the woods ever so mournful; and I heard an owl, away off, who-whooing about somebody that was dead, and a whippowill and a dog crying about somebody that was going to die; and the wind was trying to whisper something to me, and I couldn't make out what it was, and so it made the cold shivers run over me. Then away out in the woods I heard that kind of a sound that a ghost makes when it wants to tell about something that's on its mind and can't make itself understood, and so can't rest easy in its grave, and has to go about that way every night grieving. I got so down-hearted and scared I did wish I had some company. Pretty soon a spider went crawling up my shoulder, and I flipped it off and it lit in the candle; and before I could budge it was all shriveled up. I didn't need anybody to tell me that that was an awful bad sign and would fetch me some bad luck, so I was scared and most shook the clothes off of me. I got up and turned around in my tracks three times and crossed my breast every time; and then I tied up a little lock of my hair with a thread to keep witches away. But I hadn't no confidence. You do that when you've lost a horseshoe that you've found, instead of nailing it up over the door, but I hadn't ever heard anybody say it was any way to keep off bad luck when you'd killed a spider.

I set down again, a-shaking all over, and got out my pipe for a smoke; for the house was all as still as death now, and so the widow wouldn't know. Well, after a long time I heard the clock away off in the town go boom—boom—boom—twelve licks; and all still again—stiller than ever. Pretty soon I heard a twig snap down in the dark amongst the trees—something was a stirring. I set still and listened. Directly I could just barely hear a "me-yow! me-yow!" down there. That was good! Says I, "me-yow! me-yow!" as soft as I could, and then I put out the light and scrambled out of the window on to the shed. Then I slipped down to the ground and crawled in among the trees, and, sure enough, there was Tom Sawyer waiting for me.

END.

VISUAL NEGLECT

Reading Maps

Use the maps and directions to navigate.

VISUAL NEGLECT

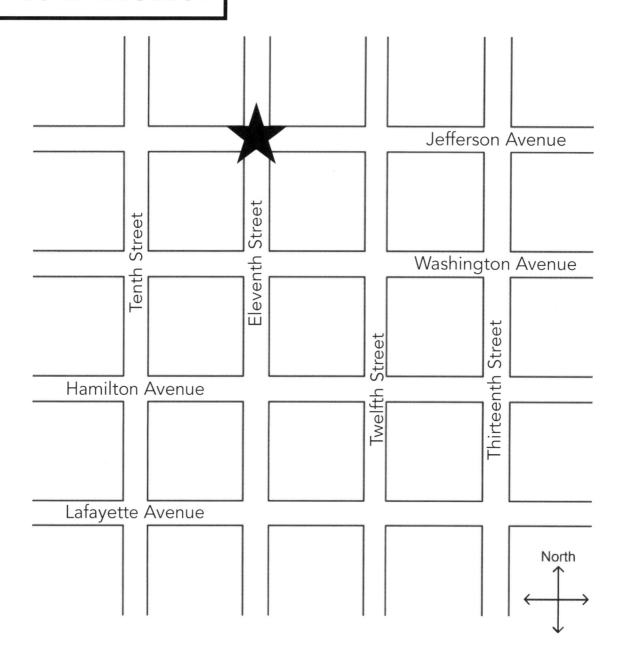

1. Start at the intersection of Jefferson Ave and Eleventh St.

2. Go South two blocks.

3. Go West one block.

4. Go South one block.

5. Where are you now? _____

VISUAL NEGLECT

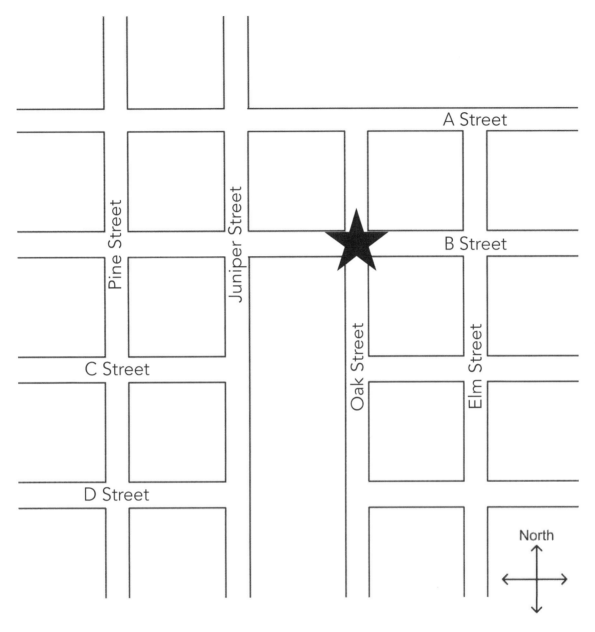

1. Start at the intersection of Oak and B St.
2. Go North one block.
3. Go West two blocks.
4. Go South three blocks.
5. Go East one block.
6. Where are you now?_____

VISUAL NEGLECT

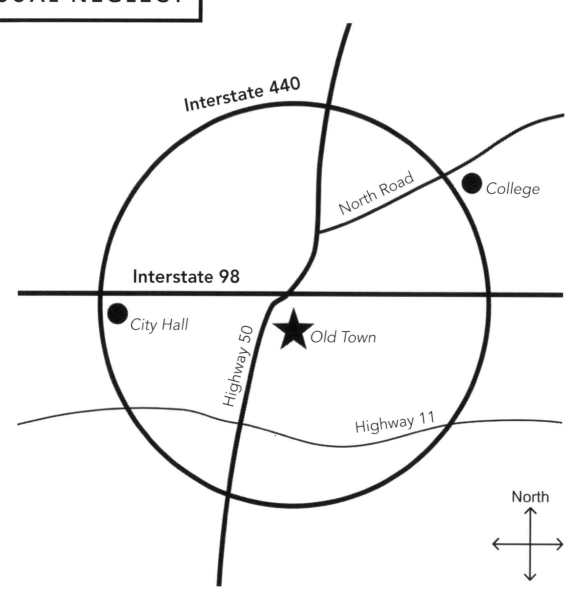

1. Start at Old Town.

2. Go North on Highway 50.

3. Which road branches off from Highway 50?

4. Go West on Interstate 440.

5. Drive until you reach Interstate 98.

6. What landmark is close by?_____

VISUAL NEGLECT

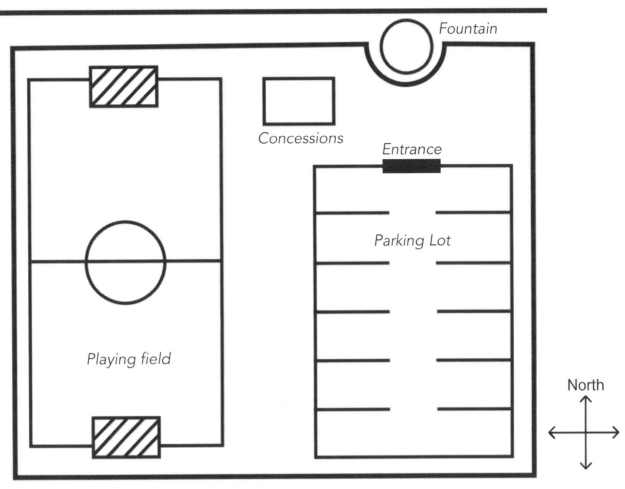

1. What road runs North of the playing field? _____

2. Is the fountain on the north side of the park? _____

3. Where is the playing field in relation to the fountain? _____

4. Which direction would I need to walk to get from the parking lot to the concession stand? _____

5. What end of the parking lot is the Entrance located? _____

VISUAL NEGLECT

Page 1 of 2

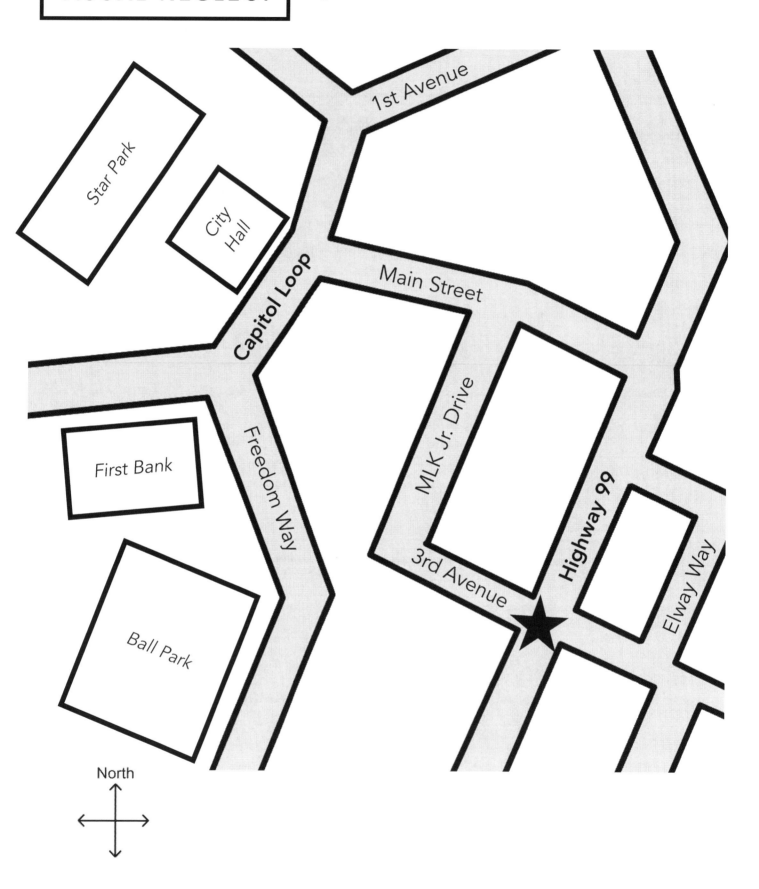

VISUAL NEGLECT

Page 2 of 2

1. Start at Highway 99 and 3rd Ave.

2. Go North on Highway 99.

3. Take the first left.

4. What landmark is at the end of the road? _____

5. Turn left again.

6. Stop at the first intersection. What landmark is on the corner?

   _____

7. What intersection are you at? _____

VISUAL NEGLECT

Page 1 of 2

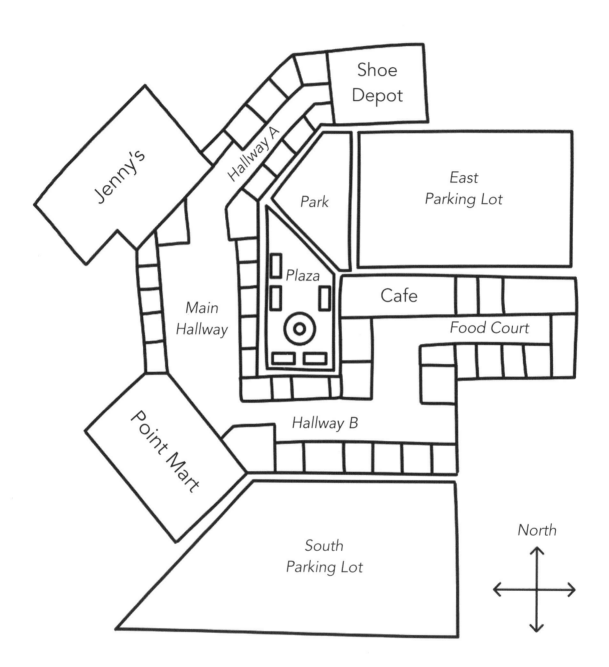

VISUAL NEGLECT

1. How do you reach the Food Court from Jenny's?

2. Is Shoe Depot near the East Parking Lot?

3. What is the southern most store?

4. Where is the park in relation to the Cafe?

5. How do you reach Shoe Depot from Point Mart?

APHASIA

Aphasia is a language disorder that affects a person's ability to produce language, understand language, or both. The goal of aphasia treatment is to increase communication effectiveness. Choose aphasia goals and techniques based on the patient's previous and current levels of functioning, amount of support available, motivation, insight into deficits, and other factors. Many patients with aphasia also benefit from support groups.

Language treatment includes:
- Restorative treatment (e.g. increasing naming ability)
- Compensatory treatment (e.g. teaching comprehension techniques to caregivers)
- Communication partner education and training (e.g. using communication strategies)
- AAC and other modalities
- Identifying the need for accommodations (e.g. receiving verbal plus written information after a medical appointment)

APHASIA

Therapist Instructions

EVALUATIONS.
- Formal batteries include the *Assessment of Language-Related Functional Activities*, *Western Aphasia Battery*, and *Boston Diagnostic Aphasia Examination*.
- Informal cognitive-linguistic evaluations often have sections covering language expression, comprehension, reading, and writing. ASHA's *Adult Language/Cognitive-Communication Evaluation* is free online (ASHA, 2021d).

DAY ONE OF TREATMENT. Provide the following handouts, as needed:
- Homework Log, Monthly Calendar, Language Impairments, Word Finding Tips, Communication Tips, Increasing Comprehension
- Highlight key points on the handouts, then review with your patients. Ask questions to make sure they understand the content. Answer any questions they may have.

FOR THERAPIST EYES ONLY. Pages marked with a gray background or header are resources for therapists. Some caregivers and patients may benefit from having a copy.
- Cueing Hierarchy, Treatment Approaches

SUPPORT GROUPS. Many people with aphasia benefit greatly from interacting with others with the same disorder. Local universities and hospitals often have aphasia groups: Call the speech therapy department for more information.

STRATEGIES. Choose 2-3 of the most useful word finding strategies and focus on those with your patient. Have these handouts available each session and refer to them often.
- Word Finding Tips, Communication Tips for expressive and receptive aphasia, Increasing Comprehension

WHITEBOARDS. Many receptive and expressive tasks in this book can be completed using a whiteboard. Patients may benefit from the larger print and ability to erase

APHASIA

easily. Transfer the material (e.g., word web, single words, phrase identification, etc.) to a handheld whiteboard.

AUDITORY PRESENTATION. These pages are marked with a gray header and are meant for you to read aloud to the patient. Some patients will benefit from having a written copy instead. Use your clinical judgment to decide what's best for your patient.
- Pages 320–329, 351–367, 378, and 388–394.

ONE-SIDED PRINTING (PAGES 399–426). Some tasks include two pages: one with reading material and the other with questions. Print these one-sided (so the patient doesn't need to flip the paper back and forth).

COPY & CUT. Copy these pages then cut along the lines:
- VNeST flashcards (page 303), word webs (page 308), Treatment of Underlying Forms flashcards (page 310), Naming Game (page 342), Identify Pictures and Words (page 369), Picture Description (page 428)

LANGUAGE ACTIVITY RESOURCE KIT (LARK). The LARK *(Dressler, 2005)* is an excellent treatment kit for patients with moderate to severe aphasia. It includes 25 objects with matching word cards and action cards. The kit is available for purchase on the publisher's website: See proedinc.com for more details.

TALKING POINTS.
- With any patient, consider the task modality (how you present the question) and the patient's response modality. You may talk/listen, read/write, or both. Use whatever modality(ies) will help your patient communicate successfully.
- Use material in the patient's environment, like greeting cards or magazines.
- Complete treatment in different environments beyond the therapy room, like the cafeteria, local coffee shop, on the phone, and with different people.

APHASIA

Contents

Cueing Hierarchy………………………..	301
Treatment Approaches…………………….	302
VNeST Flashcards………………….	303
VNeST Agent/Patient Pairs…………	307
Semantic Feature Analysis…………..	308
Phonologic Component Analysis….	309
Treatment of Underlying Forms…….	310
Language Impairments……………………..	311
Word Finding Tips……..……………………	312
Communication Tips *(Expression)*…………	313
Communication Tips *(Comprehension)*……	314
Increasing Comprehension…………………	315

LANGUAGE EXPRESSION

Alphabet………………………………….	317
Automatic Phrases……………………….	318
Object Naming……………………………	320
Sentence Completion……………………	321
Naming from Description…………………..	323
Category Naming…………………………	325
Category Members……………………….	328
Rhyming Words…………………………..	330
Same Letter………………………………..	332
Parts of a Whole………………………….	334
Same Meaning……………………………	336
Synonyms………………………………….	337
Opposite Meaning……………………….	339
Antonyms………………………………….	340

APHASIA

Naming Game………………………………..	342
Needed Items……………………………..	344
Complete the Series………………………….	347
Associated Words………………………..	348
Naming Emotions…………………………	351
Question Game……………………………..	352
Sentences………………………………..	353
Giving Directions…………………………..	355
Differences Between Words……………….	356
Definitions………………………………..	357
Conversations……………………………..	358

LANGUAGE COMPREHENSION

Body Part Identification…………………….	362
Identify Objects……………………………..	363
1-Step Directions…………………………..	364
Simple Yes/No Questions…………………...	365
Complex Yes/No Questions………………..	366
Identify Words……………………………..	367
Identify Pictures and Words……………….	368
Word Pairs………………………..	369
Picture Pairs (line drawings)…………	371
Identify Phrases……………………………	378
Phrases & Pictures…………………………	379
Follow Written Directions………………….	381
Identify Sentences…………………………	388
Paragraphs………………………………..	389
Reading…………………………………..	395
Everyday Reading…………………………	399
Picture Description *(black/white photos)*….	427

APHASIA

SEE ALSO

Neuroplasticity.............................	24
Remembering Reading Material......	165
Neuroanatomy & Physiology..........	189
Reading Material.........................	280
Phone Calls................................	454
Conversation..............................	455
Interview....................................	456
Monologues...............................	457
Alphabet Board...........................	569
Needs Board..............................	570

APHASIA

Cueing Hierarchy

This cueing hierarchy is meant to improve language expression (Wambaugh, 2003; Abel et al., 2005). It progresses from minimal to maximal assistance. Progress to the next step only when the patient is **incorrect**. Provide feedback after each step.

---

1. Ask the patient to name the picture or object.
   - For example, the picture is of a spoon. Prompt, "This is a…"
2. Provide a **description or definition**.
   - "This is an eating utensil."
3. Provide a **sentence completion** cue.
   - "I eat soup with a…"
4. Provide a **semantically loaded sentence completion** cue.
   - "I scooped the sugar with the measuring…"
5. Provide a **non-word rhyme**.
   - "It rhymes with hoon."
6. Provide an **initial sound cue**.
   - "It starts with sss."
7. Provide a **sentence completion** using the **rhyme and initial sound cue**.
   - "The name of this picture rhymes with hoon, it is a sss…"
8. **Model** the word. Ask for repetition.
   - "This is a spoon. This is a…"

APHASIA

Treatment Approaches

Below are systematic approaches for aphasia treatment. Visit theadultspeechtherapyworkbook.com for treatment protocols and additional resources. See the following pages for templates.

VNeST. Verb Network Strengthening Treatment is a naming treatment *(Edmonds et al., 2009)* where the patient retrieves specific nouns associated with verbs.
- *For example, the verb "measure" can be paired with the nouns "carpenter" and "wood."*

SEMANTIC FEATURE ANALYSIS is a naming treatment where the patient lists semantic information about the target word and creates a word web *(Davis & Stanton, 2005)*.

PHONOLOGICAL COMPONENT ANALYSIS is a naming treatment where the patient lists phonological information about the target word and creates a word web *(Leonard et al., 2008)*.

TREATMENT OF UNDERLYING FORMS is a syntax production treatment *(Thompson & Shapiro, 2005; Anderson, 2017)*. The patient produces different sentence structures by rearranging word cards to describe pictures.
- *For example, "The boy pet the cat," is changed to, "It was the cat who was pet by the boy."*

APHASIA

Who	What
Where	When
Why	

VNeST Flashcards
Copy and cut

APHASIA

Measure	
Carpenter	Wood
Chef	Ingredients
Pharmacist	Medicine

VNeST Example "Measure" Agent/Patient Pairs
Copy and cut

APHASIA *Page 3 of 5*

Catch	
Police	Criminal
Fisherman	Fish
Passenger	Bus

VNeST Example "Catch" Agent/Patient Pairs
Copy and cut

APHASIA

Throw	
Host	Party
Pitcher	Baseball
Toddler	Tantrum

VNeST Example "Throw" Agent/Patient Pairs
Copy and cut

APHASIA

ADDITIONAL VNeST AGENT/PATIENT PAIRS.

WATCH
Lifeguard/swimmers
Audience/movie
Babysitter/child
Guard/prisoners

WRITE
Author/book
Teacher/assignment
Doctor/prescription
Donor/check

FIX
Mechanic/car
Dentist/tooth
Plumber/toilet
Electrician/light

FIGHT
Patient/cancer
Boxer/opponent
Lawyer/case
Soldier/enemy

SERVE
Waiter/dinner
Barista/coffee
Athlete/volleyball
General/military

DELIVER
Midwife/baby
Mailman/letter
Anchorman/news
Jury/verdict

CONDUCT
Engineer/train
Conductor/band
Scientist/experiment
Detective/investigation

HEAL
Time/wounds
Doctor/patient
Bandaid/scratch
Cast/bone

Semantic Feature Analysis Word Web

- Association
- Properties
- Group
- Target word/picture
- Location
- Action
- Use

Rhymes with ___

First sound ___

Another word ___

Target word/picture ___

# of syllables ___

Final sound ___

Phonological Component Analysis Word Web

APHASIA

WHO	WHAT
?	IT
WAS	BY
SEEMS	TO HAVE

Treatment of Underlying Forms Flashcards
Copy and cut

APHASIA

Language Impairments

Common language impairments include:

APHASIA. A language disorder caused by brain damage that can result in difficulty understanding language, producing language, reading, and/or writing. It does not affect intelligence.

WERNICKE'S APHASIA. Also known as "receptive aphasia." Difficulty with understanding language. Patients who present with less jargon at first tend to make better progress *(Rogalski et al., 2013)*.

BROCA'S APHASIA. Also known as "expressive aphasia." Difficulty with producing language. People with Broca's aphasia typically make fair progress, with the quickest recovery happening during the first three months after the brain injury.

GLOBAL APHASIA. Also known as "receptive and expressive aphasia." Difficulty with both understanding and producing language. Progress is typically less than the other types of aphasia especially if there is no notable progress made in the first few weeks post stroke *(Swanberg et al., 2007)*. However, some patients experience a leap in progress about six months post stroke.

APHASIA

Word Finding Tips

DESCRIBE IT.
- **Who** would use it?
- **What** does it look like?
- **Where** do you find it?
- **When** would you use it?
- **Why** would you use it?
- **How** is it used?

SYNONYM. Use a similar word.
- *For example, say **piano** instead of **organ**.*

OPPOSITE WORD. Use a word with an opposite meaning.
- *For example, say **not hot** instead of **cold**.*

GROUP OR CATEGORY. Person, place, or thing.
- *For example, the section of the store you'd find the object in.*

FIRST LETTER OR FIRST SOUND.

GESTURES. Point, act out, or play charades.

APHASIA

Communication Tips

*For the loved ones of people with **expressive** aphasia (difficulty saying the right word).*

- Give the person your full attention
    - Turn off the TV, set your phone aside, and look at their face
- Encourage the person to write, draw, or use hand gestures
- Give the person extra time to respond
- Be comfortable with silence—long pauses are okay
    - It is not necessary to fill pauses with small talk
- Avoid guessing the word or speaking for the person unless asked for help
  (National Aphasia Association, n.d.-a)
- Write down key words to improve understanding
- After the person speaks, summarize what was said and ask if you understood correctly
- Avoid "quizzing" the person—this may cause frustration
- Avoid "speaking down" to the person
    - Use simple sentences and talk slower only when needed
- Avoid speaking louder unless the person has a hearing loss
    - Aphasia does not affect hearing, so speaking loudly does not help
- If communication breaks down or the person looks frustrated or exhausted, take a break—come back to it later

| APHASIA |

Communication Tips

*For the loved ones of people with **receptive** aphasia (difficulty understanding words).*

- Give the person your full attention *(The National Aphasia Association, n.d.-b)*
    - Turn off the TV, set your phone aside, and look at their face
- Ask yes/no questions
- Get to the point and avoid extra information
- Communicate in different ways
    - Talk, pantomime, use gestures, facial expressions, pictures, and writing
- Repeat what they said then ask if you understood correctly
- Give the person extra time and be patient
- Ask them to repeat what you said
- Avoid speaking louder unless the person has a hearing loss
    - Aphasia does not affect affect hearing, so speaking loudly does not help
- Avoid pretending that you understand
    - Instead, ask them to repeat it or say it in a different way
    - Apologize for not understanding—let them know that you want to understand
- If communication breaks down or the person looks frustrated or exhausted, take a break—come back to it later

APHASIA

Increasing Comprehension

GATHER SUPPLIES. Have a writing surface and utensil ready.

WRITE THE MAIN TOPIC. In large capital letters, write the main topic of your conversation at the top of the writing surface. This will be at maximum 3 words.
- *"DOCTOR VISIT"*

WRITE KEYWORDS. Write down keywords below the main topic.
- Add bullet points to your keywords.
- Pause for a moment while your loved one reads.
    - *"BLOOD SAMPLE"*

COMMUNICATE. Say what you want to say. Use short, simple sentences.
- Avoid "talking down" to your loved one by maintaining your normal speech patterns.
    - *"You have a doctor visit on Wednesday. The doctor needs a blood sample."*

ASK QUESTIONS. Ask your loved one questions to make sure they understood your message.
- *"Why are you going to the doctor on Wednesday?"*
- *"Do I need to say it a different way?"*

APHASIA

Language Expression and Writing

APHASIA

Alphabet

Sing the alphabet song while pointing to each letter.

A B C D E F G

H I J K

L M N O P

Q R S

T U V

W X

Y Z

APHASIA

Automatic Phrases

Say each of the series aloud, pointing to each number or word as you go.

---

1 2 3 4 5 6 7 8 9 10.

10   20   30   40   50
60   70   80   90   100.

100   200   300   400   500
600   700   800   900   1,000.

APHASIA

Monday, Tuesday, Wednesday, Thursday, Friday, Saturday, Sunday.

Spring, Summer, Fall, Winter.

January, February, March, April, May, June, July, August, September, October, November, December.

Mercury, Venus, Earth, Mars, Jupiter, Saturn, Uranus, *Pluto*.

APHASIA

Object Naming

One by one, point to each physical object listed then ask the patient, "What is the name of this?" Substitute objects or use pictures as needed.

1. Chair
2. Bag
3. Remote
4. Ceiling
5. Walker
6. Table
7. Lamp
8. Pencil
9. Floor
10. Water
11. Window
12. Book
13. Papers
14. Stairs
15. Crackers
16. Door
17. Glasses
18. Phone
19. Shoes
20. Shirt
21. Sofa
22. Rug
23. Sock
24. Hair
25. Ear
26. Elbow
27. Knee
28. Shoulder
29. Fingers
30. Ring
31. Pillow
32. Keys

APHASIA

Sentence Completion

Ask the patient to complete the sentence. Either read the sentence aloud or have the patient read the sentence. They may say or write the answer.

1. This room is either too hot or too …
2. My pants are either too loose or too …
3. You are either wrong or …
4. He is either happy or …
5. The answer can be true or …
6. You can go either up or …
7. Not everything is black or …
8. I can't tell if it's day or …
9. The towel is either wet or …
10. He bought a new set of table and …
11. Do you have any brothers or …
12. It's too bright in here, please turn off the …
13. I grabbed the shampoo and washed my …

APHASIA

14. Take out the kettle and boil some …

15. She went to the library to borrow a …

16. I haven't seen you in a long …

17. You go to the bank to deposit a …

18. You have a bad headache, so you take some …

19. I fill up my car tank with …

20. I wake up at 8 …

21. I'm exhausted, so I'm going to …

22. I can't hear the TV, can you turn up the …

23. To make toast, I need one slice of …

24. I eat soup with a …

25. Pour the water into the …

26. I take coffee with cream and …

27. Take out the ice from the …

28. I placed the cake pan in the hot …

29. There are twelve months in one …

30. There are twenty-four hours in one …

31. There are seven days in one …

32. I need to lock the door with the …

33. He stopped the car at the red …

APHASIA

Naming from Description

Ask the patient to name what is being described. Either read the sentences aloud or have the patient read them. They may say or write the answer.

1. This animal is black and white, is from Africa, and looks like a horse.
2. These structures are found in Egypt, are the tombs of pharaohs, and are shaped like triangles.
3. This place is made up of islands in the Pacific Ocean and is known for ukuleles, hula skirts, and is a state in the United States.
4. This instrument is round and you use sticks to play it.
5. These are worn on your feet and are usually worn with shoes.
6. This food is typically eaten for breakfast, comes from a chicken, and can be fried, scrambled, or boiled.
7. This alcoholic drink is made from grapes, famously comes from Italy or France, and is sold in glass bottles.
8. This job involves going to court and proving people to be guilty or innocent.
9. This tool is used to cut logs in half and has "teeth."
10. This vehicle has many seats, wings, and can fly.
11. This grows in the fall, is orange, and is associated with Halloween.
12. This goes over a small wounds, sticks to your skin, and helps avoid infection.

APHASIA

13. This is driven by an engineer, transports people or goods, and runs on rails.
14. This indicates when to stop, go, or slow down while driving on the road.
15. This has eight limbs and lives in the ocean.
16. This is worn on your wrist and tells you the time.
17. This is a form of art often carved out of stone. The work "David" is a famous example.
18. This sport involves skating on ice and scoring goals using sticks and pucks.
19. This is used as a shelter for campers and is made with fabric and poles.
20. This natural disaster is measured by magnitude and relates to plate tectonics.
21. This famous painter from Italy created the Mona Lisa and was an inventor.
22. This city in Europe is known for baguettes and the Eiffel Tower.
23. This vehicle has four wheels and can be pulled by horses.
24. This is the part of the computer that you type on and has many letters and numbers on it.
25. This is a place where you can buy a ticket, wait by the tracks, and board vehicles that run on rails.
26. This event happens on the same day every year to celebrate a marriage.
27. This is the illegal action of taking someone's belongings without their permission.
28. This is the emotion you feel when you wake up to a sound in the middle of the night and you are alone.

APHASIA Page 1 of 3

Category Naming

Ask the patient to name what category each set of words belongs to. Either read the words aloud or have the patient read them. They may say or write the answer.

1. Dog, cat, horse, pig
2. Water, juice, milk, coffee
3. Spring, summer, fall, winter
4. Shirt, jeans, sweater, blouse
5. Texas, Florida, California, Alabama
6. Hammer, screwdriver, saw, wrench
7. Notepad, stapler, scissors, tape
8. New Year's Day, Mother's Day, Christmas, Halloween
9. Table, sofa, chair, bed
10. Milk, yogurt, cheese, creamer
11. Pie, cake, ice cream, tart
12. December, January, February, March
13. Maple, cedar, oak, birch
14. Red, blue, yellow, green
15. Apple, pear, plum, banana

APHASIA

16. Happy, sad, angry, scared
17. Slippers, socks, boots, shoes
18. Bacon, waffles, eggs, hash-browns
19. Cinnamon, pepper, paprika, nutmeg
20. Dishwasher, oven, refrigerator, microwave
21. Gloves, scarf, hat, mittens
22. Hot, warm, cool, cold
23. Corn, potato, carrot, radish
24. Sweet, sour, salty, bitter
25. Morning, night, dawn, dusk
26. Plate, cup, bowl, saucer
27. China, South Korea, Japan, Thailand
28. Ferry, yacht, canoe, kayak
29. Lipstick, mascara, blush, eyeliner
30. Rainy, sunny, cloudy, snowy
31. Library, bank, grocery store, café
32. Drama, romance, action, comedy
33. Hinduism, Catholicism, Judaism, Buddhism
34. Duck, swan, seagull, heron
35. Trout, carp, salmon, tuna

APHASIA

36. Broom, bleach, mop, sponge
37. Mercury, Venus, Earth, Mars
38. English, Math, Philosophy, Art
39. Strawberries, cherries, raspberries, pomegranates
40. Chicago, London, Sydney, Toronto
41. Kite, airplane, bird, helicopter
42. Chamomile, green, black, earl grey
43. Blue, orca, humpback, beluga
44. Quarter, penny, dime, nickel
45. Glossary, chapter, introduction, table of contents
46. Ham, bacon, ribs, loin
47. Washington, Kennedy, Lincoln, Bush
48. Anne, Elizabeth, Victoria, Mary
49. Teal, cyan, navy, sky
50. Granny Smith, Red Delicious, Mcintosh, Honeycrisp
51. Keyboard, mouse, monitor, speakers
52. Arctic, ice, freezer, snowflake
53. Times, Herald, Daily, Gazette
54. Saxophone, tuba, trumpet, trombone
55. Yield, merge, stop, turn

APHASIA

Category Members

Ask the patient to name 3 or more items that belong to each category. Or ask them to name as many items from each category as they can in 1 minute. Either read the categories aloud or have the patient read them. They may say or write the answers.

ANIMALS.
- Farm animals
- Jungle animals
- Rodents
- Carnivores
- Herbivores

FOODS.
- Breakfast foods
- Meat
- Vegetables
- Fruits
- Salty foods

BEVERAGES.
- Hot beverages
- Cold beverages
- Alcoholic beverages
- Kid beverages
- Carbonated beverages

PLACES.
- Cities
- Countries
- Tourist attractions
- Bodies of water
- Ancient places

HOUSEHOLD OBJECTS.
- Kitchen objects
- Furniture
- Bedroom objects
- Bathroom objects
- Lawn and garden objects

PEOPLE'S NAMES.
- Men's names
- Women's names
- Last names
- Family member names
- Names that start with "S"

CLOTHING.
- Cold weather clothing
- Hot weather clothing
- Formal clothing

STORES.
- Restaurants
- Clothing stores
- Big-box retail stores

SPORTS.
- Olympic sports
- Sports played with a ball
- Individual sports

IMPORTANT EVENTS.
- Holidays
- Wars
- Award shows

PROFESSIONS.
- Healthcare professions
- Blue collar jobs
- Technology jobs

MUSICAL INSTRUMENTS.
- String instruments
- Woodwind instruments
- Popular musical instruments

ACTIVITIES.
- Hobbies
- Household chores
- Vacation activities

ENTERTAINMENT.
- TV Shows
- Movies
- Musicians/Bands

APHASIA — Page 1 of 2

Rhyming Words

Fill in the blank with the word that is being described. All of the answers rhyme with each other.

---

1. Past tense of "spin" _____

2. What Earth revolves around _____

3. You put a hotdog in it _____

3. 2,000 pounds equals one _____

4. A religious woman _____

5. Granddaughter's brother _____

6. Enjoyable and entertaining _____

7. More than zero _____

8. More than a jog _____

9. Avoid or reject someone _____

10. Opposite of lose _____

APHASIA

11. Not any _____

12. A loud weapon _____

13. No longer happening _____

15. Past tense of "begin" _____

16. Shock or amaze _____

17. Nineteen plus two _____

18. Cooked too much _____

20. Word play or a joke _____

APHASIA

Same Letter

Fill in the blank with the word that is being described. All of the answers begin with the same letter.

---

1. A feline pet　　　　　　　　　　_____

2. Automobile with four wheels　　_____

3. You drink out of one　　　　　　_____

4. You sit on it by a table　　　　　_____

5. A large town　　　　　　　　　　_____

6. A dessert topped with icing　　　_____

7. Similar to a sofa　　　　　　　　_____

8. 100 years　　　　　　　　　　　_____

9. Given out on Halloween　　　　　_____

10. Replicate or imitate　　　　　　_____

APHASIA

11. A producer of milk   _____

12. Coins and bills   _____

13. What rabbits eat   _____

14. A professional cook   _____

15. A baby cow   _____

16. An accessory for your head   _____

17. An animal that crosses deserts   _____

18. Like a walking stick   _____

19. Opposite of stormy   _____

20. Zoo animals live in these   _____

APHASIA

Parts of a Whole

Each word listed is a part of a whole. For example, Wheels are part of a Car. Say or write each answer in the blank spaces. There may be more than one correct answer.

1. Wheels are part of a _____Car_____

2. Months _____

3. Pages _____

4. Icing _____

5. Bones _____

6. Keyboard _____

7. Bathroom _____

8. Teeth _____

9. Fingers _____

10. Motor _____

APHASIA

Page 2 of 2

11. Afternoon _____

12. Mother _____

13. Australia _____

14. Chorus _____

15. Yellow _____

16. Legs _____

17. Drain _____

18. Wednesday _____

19. Strings _____

20. Infancy _____

21. Ink _____

APHASIA

Same Meaning

Read each target word. Then, select the two words with the same/similar meaning.

1. Bad	☐ Awful	☐ Terrible
	☐ Large	☐ Average
2. Good	☐ Funny	☐ Great
	☐ Excellent	☐ Enough
3. Move	☐ Front	☐ Go
	☐ Back	☐ Hurry
4. Sad	☐ Mad	☐ Short
	☐ Unhappy	☐ Gloomy
5. Say	☐ Tell	☐ Know
	☐ Truth	☐ Explain
6. Old	☐ Young	☐ Ancient
	☐ Aged	☐ Deep
7. Interesting	☐ Fascinating	☐ Boring
	☐ Long	☐ Intriguing
8. Fast	☐ Food	☐ Angry
	☐ Quick	☐ Speedy
9. Beautiful	☐ Kind	☐ Gorgeous
	☐ Sunrise	☐ Pretty

APHASIA

Synonyms

Read each word. Say or write in a similar word; a word that has the same meaning.

---

1. Begin _____

2. Funny _____

3. Beautiful _____

4. Finish _____

5. Small _____

6. Hot _____

7. Good _____

8. Dull _____

9. Smart _____

10. Difficult _____

11. Big _____

12. Young _____

13. Fast _____

14. Mad _____

15. Happy _____

16. Purchase _____

APHASIA

17. Bottom

    _____

18. Top

    _____

19. Shout

    _____

20. Sick

    _____

21. Gift

    _____

22. Baby

    _____

23. Talk

    _____

24. Fix

    _____

25. Help

    _____

26. Give

    _____

27. Break

    _____

28. Easy

    _____

29. Many

    _____

30. Low

    _____

31. Make

    _____

32. Superior

    _____

33. Noisy

    _____

34. Quiet

    _____

35. Busy

    _____

36. Shy

    _____

37. Believe

    _____

38. Amazing

    _____

APHASIA

Opposite Meaning

Read each target word. Then, select the two words with the opposite meaning.

1. Begin	☐ Slow ☐ End	☐ Finish ☐ Middle
2. Hot	☐ Icy ☐ Cold	☐ Humid ☐ Summer
3. Love	☐ Like ☐ Enjoy	☐ Hate ☐ Detest
4. Small	☐ Huge ☐ Petite	☐ Large ☐ Light
5. Light	☐ Measure ☐ Skinny	☐ Dark ☐ Heavy
6. Easy	☐ Difficult ☐ Hard	☐ Meeting ☐ Simple
7. Slow	☐ Quick ☐ Steady	☐ Move ☐ Fast
8. Fun	☐ Place ☐ Boring	☐ Time ☐ Dull
9. Sad	☐ Horrible ☐ Dreadful	☐ Cheerful ☐ Joyful

APHASIA

Antonyms

Read each word. Say or write in an opposite word; a word with the opposite meaning.

---

1. Inside
   _____

2. Freezing
   _____

3. No
   _____

4. Good
   _____

5. Early
   _____

6. Tired
   _____

7. Going
   _____

8. Positive
   _____

9. Up
   _____

10. Sweet
    _____

11. Open
    _____

12. Left
    _____

13. Above
    _____

14. Day
    _____

15. Bottom
    _____

16. Terrible
    _____

APHASIA

17. Ugly
   _____

18. White
   _____

19. Busy
   _____

20. Pleased
   _____

21. Careful
   _____

22. Outside
   _____

23. Deny
   _____

24. Increase
   _____

25. Best
   _____

26. Fix
   _____

27. Refuse
   _____

28. Accurate
   _____

29. Against
   _____

30. Never
   _____

31. Awake
   _____

32. Spend
   _____

33. Combine
   _____

34. Sunrise
   _____

35. Kill
   _____

36. Go
   _____

37. Borrow
   _____

38. Depressed
   _____

APHASIA

Naming Game

Copy then cut out each game card. Play this game with two people or two groups. The goal of the game is to have the other person/group guess the **BOLD** word at the top of each box. You can't say any of the words written in that box. Instead, use synonyms, antonyms, or describe the word using full sentences. You can also "talk around" the word and use gestures.

VIOLIN Instrument Strings Viola	**RASPBERRY** Berry Red Pie	**CUCUMBER** Zucchini Green Vegetable
FORD Car Motor Truck	**TOOTHBRUSH** Teeth Toothpaste Floss	**REMOTE** Television Channel Volume
ROSE Flower Bud Smell	**MAILBOX** Letter Package Mailman	**FINGERNAIL** Scratch Polish Fingers

APHASIA

HAPPY Feeling Good Sad	**BIRTHDAY** Year Old Age	**JUMP** Up Down Hop
COLLEGE School University Degree Credits	**SUMMER** Warm Hot Sun Beach	**SUPERMAN** Cape Superhero Clark Kent Lois Lane
NEW YORK City Times Square Big Apple Statue of Liberty	**WRITING** Letter Pen Paper Note	**DOCTOR** Nurse Hospital Physician Prescription
UNDER Beneath Over Down Top	**NAPKIN** Tissue Kleenex Paper Towel Clean	**TRAVELING** Going Vacation Airplane Car

APHASIA

Needed Items

Name three items you need to...

---

1. Make a cup of tea

   _____   _____   _____

2. Make a peanut butter and jelly sandwich

   _____   _____   _____

3. Fry an egg

   _____   _____   _____

4. Cook pasta

   _____   _____   _____

5. Make a salad

   _____   _____   _____

6. Go on a camping trip

   _____   _____   _____

APHASIA

7. Make a holiday dinner

8. Plant a seed

9. Change a tire

10. Clean a bathroom

11. Clean a car

12. Go on a road trip

13. Renew a passport

14. Hire a plumber

APHASIA

15. Travel by airplane

    _____   _____   _____

16. Get a new job

    _____   _____   _____

17. Throw a birthday party

    _____   _____   _____

18. Raise a puppy

    _____   _____   _____

19. Make a flower bouquet

    _____   _____   _____

20. Construct a house

    _____   _____   _____

APHASIA

Complete the Series

Add a word that logically follows.

1. First, second, third, _____

2. Seed, sprout, sapling, _____

3. Wednesday, Thursday, Friday, _____

4. Summer, Fall, Winter, _____

5. Infant, toddler, child, _____

6. A, B, C, _____

7. Ten, eleven, twelve, _____

8. Freshman, sophomore, junior, _____

9. Red, orange, yellow, _____

10. Mercury, Venus, Earth, _____

11. Cold, cool, warm, _____

12. Extra large, large, medium, _____

13. Dawn, day, dusk, _____

14. Larva, caterpillar, cocoon, _____

15. Horse, wagon, train, _____

16. Puddle, pond, lake, _____

APHASIA

Associated Words

For each word listed, name three words that you associate with it. For example, "Cat: fur, kitten, meow." There are many correct answers.

---

1. Doctor
   _____ _____ _____

2. Artist
   _____ _____ _____

3. Engineer
   _____ _____ _____

4. Mechanic
   _____ _____ _____

5. Teacher
   _____ _____ _____

6. Witch
   _____ _____ _____

7. Fisherman
   _____ _____ _____

8. Mailman
   _____ _____ _____

APHASIA

9. Politician

   _____   _____   _____

10. Queen

    _____   _____   _____

11. President

    _____   _____   _____

12. Judge

    _____   _____   _____

13. Grandma

    _____   _____   _____

14. Dinner

    _____   _____   _____

15. Morning

    _____   _____   _____

16. Birthday

    _____   _____   _____

17. Vacation

    _____   _____   _____

18. Wilderness

    _____   _____   _____

19. Baking

    _____   _____   _____

APHASIA

20. Childhood

21. Courage

22. Festival

23. Math

24. Career

25. Tradition

26. Leisure

27. Patriot

28. Earth

29. Universe

30. Choice

APHASIA

Naming Emotions

Ask the patient, "How would you feel in the following situations? What emotions would you feel?"

1. You got your dream job.
2. All of your loved ones forgot your birthday.
3. A person yells at you and calls you bad names.
4. You hear on the news that your hometown experienced a natural disaster.
5. Your good friend has a baby.
6. You are driving and see a police car with its lights on right behind you.
7. The political candidate you voted for loses the election.
8. You worked hard all day and now you're taking a hot bath.
9. The neighbor's dog barks at 4 am, waking you up.
10. You drive to your very last day of work and retire tomorrow.
11. You wait for the doctor for over an hour and your appointment lasts 5 minutes.
12. Your friends throw you a surprise birthday party.
13. Your insurance company tells you that they will not cover your recent surgery.
14. You win a raffle prize worth $1,000.
15. You are offered a free, all-expenses-paid trip to the moon.
16. You are waiting to hear back from the doctor about the test results.
17. You get laid off the day before you're eligible for a pension.
18. You are in a store, you have a headache, and it is very crowded.

APHASIA

Question Game

Have your patient guess each word. They can ask you up to 20 'yes' or 'no' questions. If they struggle to come up with questions, model the activity: Share the answer and ask yes/no questions for them.

1. Napoleon Bonaparte
2. The Great Wall of China
3. Mount Everest
4. Hawaii
5. Martin Luther King, Jr.
6. Bathroom
7. Jesus Christ
8. Alaska
9. Valentine's Day
10. Pumpkin
11. Marilyn Monroe
12. Nurse
13. Movie theater
14. New Year's Day
15. The bank
16. Seat belt
17. The Beatles
18. Playground
19. Gold
20. Dracula
21. Mother Teresa
22. Egyptian Pyramids
23. Sherlock Holmes
24. Buddha
25. Piano
26. Chopsticks
27. California
28. Australia
29. Hammer
30. Queen Elizabeth
31. Ice cube
32. Lightning
33. Oprah Winfrey
34. Frida Kahlo
35. Cleopatra
36. Lawn mower

APHASIA

Sentences

Read the following scenarios aloud to your patient. Your patient will fill in the blanks.

1. You're at a restaurant and your salad arrives. You realize you don't have any utensils. You turn to your waiter and say…

2. You are at the movie theatre. The person sitting next to you is talking so loudly that you can't hear the movie. You turn to the person and say…

3. You are at the shopping mall and see a little girl standing all alone. She is crying and looking around for someone. You approach the little girl and say…

4. Your doctor appointment starts in 10 minutes, but you are stuck in traffic. You call up the doctor's office and say…

5. You find a pair of glasses on the ground. A few minutes later, you see someone squinting, searching the ground, and patting his pockets. You approach him and say…

6. You are shopping for shoes and find a pair you like. After looking, you realize they don't have your size. You approach the store worker and say…

APHASIA

7. You go to the bank with your paycheck. You approach the teller, hand over the check, and say…

8. You call the pizza restaurant to order dinner for your family. The worker answers and you say…

9. You are paying for groceries with a check, but you are not sure what the date is. You ask the cashier…

10. You are leaving a store, but someone is speaking on the phone and blocking the exit. You say to the person…

11. You are at a restaurant looking at the menu. The server asks what you'd like to eat, but you haven't decided yet. You say to the server…

12. You look outside and see a strange dog in your backyard. A few minutes later, you hear your neighbor calling a dog's name. You go outside and say to your neighbor…

13. You arrive at the large building for your appointment with a specialist. You do not see a directory. You approach the receptionist and say…

14. You are at the deli counter and ask for a half-pound of ham. The deli worker starts cutting some turkey. You say to the worker…

APHASIA

Giving Directions

Ask your patient to describe how to do each activity in as much detail as possible. "Pretend that I've never done these activities before. How do I...?"

1. Brush my teeth
2. Make a cup of tea
3. Boil a pot of water
4. Mail a letter
5. Make toast
6. Deposit a check
7. Do a jumping jack
8. Peel a banana
9. Plant a seed
10. Fold a shirt
11. Wash a car
12. Order at a fast-food restaurant
13. Make a snowman
14. Do the laundry
15. Make a grilled cheese sandwich
16. Wash my hair
17. Make a paper airplane
18. Return an item to the store
19. Hammer in a nail
20. Roast a marshmallow
21. Ask a stranger for directions
22. Clean up broken glass from the floor
23. Change a light bulb
24. Make a cup of hot chocolate
25. Start a fire
26. Pay a credit card bill
27. Tie my shoes
28. Put on gloves
29. Clean up spilled milk
30. Reach something on a high shelf
31. Make ice cubes
32. Navigate a new building
33. Book a hotel room
34. Use a calculator
35. Rent a movie
36. Refill my prescription

APHASIA

Differences Between Words

Ask the patient, "What is the difference between these two words?" There are many correct answers.

1. Lock and key
2. Flowers and grass
3. Ketchup and mustard
4. Guitar and violin
5. Spoon and fork
6. Coffee and tea
7. Newspaper and magazine
8. Bracelet and necklace
9. Honey and syrup
10. Bread and toast
11. Rock and pebble
12. Bookstore and library
13. Bicycle and motorcycle
14. Bronze and gold
15. Small and minuscule
16. Sluggish and slow
17. Tissue and napkin
18. Sandwich and taco
19. Crib and bed
20. Leaf and petal
21. Ocean and sea
22. Sweater and jacket
23. Shoe and boot
24. Wool and leather
25. Chicken and turkey
26. Push and shove
27. Fire and heater
28. Country and continent
29. Chair and sofa
30. Pen and marker
31. Pot and pan
32. Walk and pace
33. Sympathy and empathy
34. Excited and anxious

APHASIA

Definitions

Ask your patient to define each word, adding as much detail as possible. "Pretend that I'm from another planet. What is (a)…?"

1. Summertime
2. Calendar
3. Globe
4. Friendship
5. University
6. Gold
7. Nod
8. Photo album
9. Soda can
10. Jealousy
11. Greeting card
12. Handshake
13. Helicopter
14. Airplane
15. Sandwich
16. Taco
17. Speech therapist
18. Goal
19. Moon
20. Microwave
21. Shopping mall
22. Frustration
23. Relaxation
24. Leather
25. Lawnmower
26. Sunrise
27. Hiking
28. Wheelbarrow
29. Dreaming
30. Yesterday
31. Royalty
32. Cemetery
33. Elevator
34. Appointment
35. Challenging
36. Mailbox

APHASIA

Conversations

Ask the patient, "What would you do if…" Encourage them to add as much detail of possible.

1. You inherited a million dollars
2. You could go to university for free
3. You could fly
4. You were a famous celebrity
5. You were the President of the United States
6. You never had to sleep again
7. You knew the world was going to end in 3 days
8. You were 25 again
9. You were invisible
10. You could travel anywhere in the world
11. Your touch turned things into gold
12. You could teach any subject
13. You were at a bank and armed robbers came in
14. You found treasure in your backyard
15. You were sentenced to life in prison
16. You could travel back in time to any major event
17. You could renovate your house however you wished
18. An alien showed up at your front door
19. You lived for 100 more years
20. The stock market crashed

APHASIA

Conversations

Ask your patient to include as much detail in their answers as possible.

1. What is your favorite season and why?
2. What is your favorite sporting event and why?
3. What is your favorite type of vacation and why?
4. What was your first job?
5. What was your favorite job and why?
6. How are you similar to your parents? How are you different from your parents?
7. What is your favorite thing about yourself and why?
8. Who is your favorite person and why?
9. You can travel back in time. What time and place do you travel to and why?
10. Where was your favorite place to live and why?
11. Describe the best day you've ever had.
12. Describe your earliest memory.
13. What do you want to be remembered for?
14. What five things would you bring to a desert island and why?
15. Coffee or tea? Why?
16. What is your proudest achievement?
17. What is the worst natural disaster you lived through?
18. What is your favorite family tradition?
19. What is the thing that people are most surprised to learn about you?

APHASIA

Conversations

Ask your patient, "Would you rather…" Encourage them to add as much detail of possible.

1. Live 100 years ago or 100 years from now? Why?
2. Have an extra hand or an extra foot? Why?
3. Have $1,000 now or $2,000 in one year? Why?
4. Adopt a puppy or an adult dog? Why?
5. Eat the same thing everyday or only drink smoothies? Why?
6. Have an extra long summer or extra long winter? Why?
7. Be 6" shorter or 6" taller? Why?
8. Have a tiny apartment in the middle of a major city or a huge mansion in the country? Why?
9. Have the ability to speak with animals or read other people's minds? Why?
10. Have too many friends or too few? Why?
11. Have the ability to fly or breathe underwater? Why?
12. Go skydiving or bungee jumping? Why?
13. Spend a year in the Amazon or the outback? Why?
14. That it rain spaghetti or crackers? Why?
15. Drive a motorcycle or a dump truck everywhere? Why?
16. Have free airplane tickets for a year or free utility bills for a year? Why?
17. Have a tail or fur? Why?

APHASIA

Language Comprehension and Reading

APHASIA

Body Part Identification

Say: "Point to your…"

1. Nose
2. Ear
3. Knee
4. Stomach
5. Shoulder
6. Cheek
7. Head
8. Elbow
9. Foot
10. Neck
11. Forehead
12. Heart
13. Eyebrow
14. Chest
15. Chin
16. Lips
17. Thigh
18. Ankle
19. Temple
20. Shin

APHASIA

Identify Objects

Say: "Point to the..." Skip or substitute objects as needed.

1. Chair
2. Bag
3. Remote
4. Ceiling
5. Walker
6. Table
7. Lamp
8. Pencil
9. Floor
10. Water
11. Window
12. Book
13. Papers
14. Stairs
15. Crackers
16. Door
17. Glasses
18. Phone
19. Shoes
20. Shirt
21. Sofa
22. Rug
23. Sock
24. Hair
25. Ear
26. Elbow
27. Knee
28. Shoulder
29. Fingers
30. Ring
31. Pillow
32. Keys

APHASIA

1-Step Directions

Have a pencil and piece of paper ready. If neither are available, substitute any two objects that are easy to pick up, such as a remote or book.

1. Raise your hand
2. Raise your eyebrows
3. Clap your hands
4. Shrug your shoulders
5. Smile
6. Point to the floor
7. Give a thumbs up
8. Pick up the pencil
9. Turn over the paper
10. Put the pencil on the paper
11. Point to the window with the pencil
12. Raise your left foot
13. Tap the ground three times with your right foot
14. Blink twice
15. Hold the paper over your head
16. Touch your head with your left hand
17. Wave using both hands
18. Touch your right knee with your right hand
19. Move the pencil from your right hand to your left hand
20. Hold up three fingers

APHASIA

Simple Yes/No Questions

1. Is this month December?
2. Are you 40 years old?
3. Are you wearing shoes?
4. Do you live in California?
5. Do you have two daughters?
6. Are you wearing a hat?
7. Are you sitting in a chair?
8. Do you own a phone?
9. Is it the weekend?
10. Is it cloudy outside?
11. Are you a man?
12. Is your shirt black?
13. Is it morning time?
14. Is this season summer?
15. Is this a metal chair?
16. Are you wearing glasses?
17. Did you eat dinner yet?
18. Do you own a TV?
19. Do you have any sons?
20. Are you wearing socks?

APHASIA

Complex Yes/No

1. Do you put on your shoes and then your socks?
2. Do you bake a cake and then put on the frosting?
3. Do you make it on time if you are 10 minutes late?
4. Do you drive away and then start the car?
5. Is an ant larger than a mouse?
6. Is 30 more than 20?
7. Is day darker than night?
8. Is fire colder than ice?
9. Does Monday come before Friday?
10. Is 6 pm earlier than 3 pm?
11. Do seven days equal one week?
12. Do carrots come from a tree?
13. Do you eat soup with a spoon?
14. Do you turn on the air conditioning to cool down?
15. Does winter include January?
16. Does 11 come before 10?
17. Is a yard longer than a foot?
18. Is a decade longer than a century?
19. Do you save more money with 50% off than 30% off?
20. Do you eat cereal with a knife?
21. Do you celebrate New Year's Day in the summer?
22. Do you add ice to make a drink colder?

APHASIA

Identify Words

Write down a pair of words on a whiteboard, then say one of the words aloud. Ask the patient to point to the word you said. Erase then write the next pair of words.

1. bed — rest
2. sock — shoe
3. doctor — nurse
4. soup — salad
5. happy — angry
6. spring — summer
7. week — year
8. cold — hot
9. rain — pain
10. phone — paper
11. bowl — plate
12. door — open
13. brush — fork
14. chair — sofa
15. sink — bath
16. towel — slippers
17. shirt — sweater
18. yes — no
19. off — on
20. Sunday — Friday

APHASIA

Identify Pictures and Words

1. Copy then cut out the following word cards and picture cards.
2. Place **two pictures** in front of the patient.
3. Add **one word card** that matches one of the pictures.
4. Say the word aloud.
5. Ask the patient to point to the picture that matches that word.

You may also place **two words cards** and **one picture** in front of the patient then ask which word matches the picture.

To simplify: Place **two pictures** (or two words) in front of the patient. Without placing down a matching card, say the name of one of them. Ask the patient to point to the matching card.

hand	foot
chair	sofa
heart	star
horse	cow
hammer	screwdriver
glove	sock
motorcycle	bicycle
zebra	giraffe
clock	calendar
lion	tiger

sandwich	burger
knife	scissors
leaf	flower
banana	corn
rocket	airplane
umbrella	hat
mug	bowl
lock	key
wagon	wheelbarrow
up	down

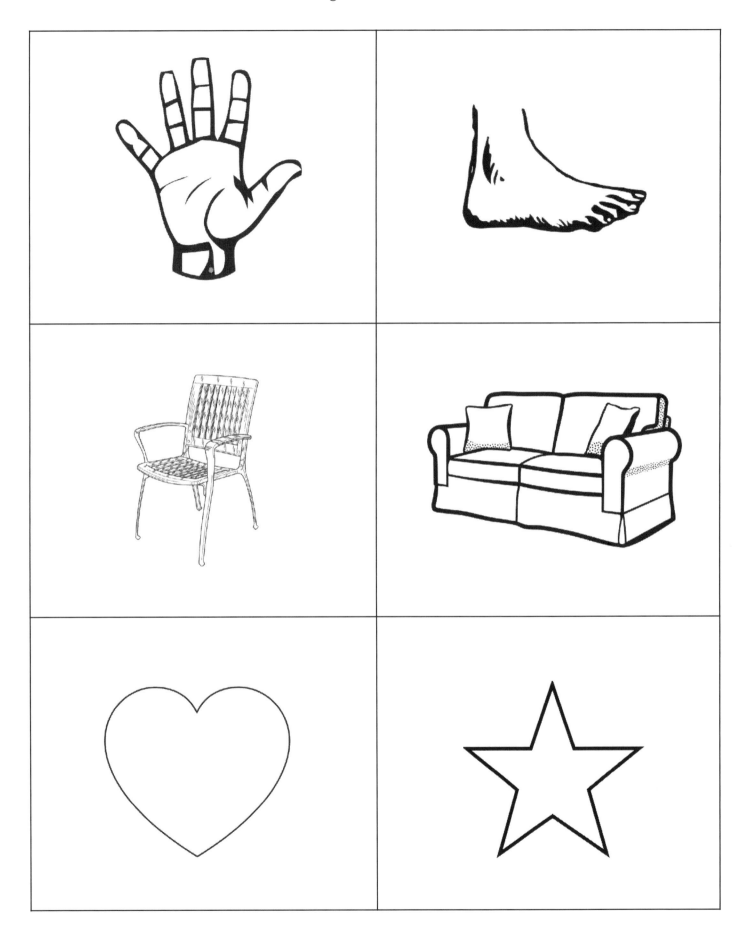

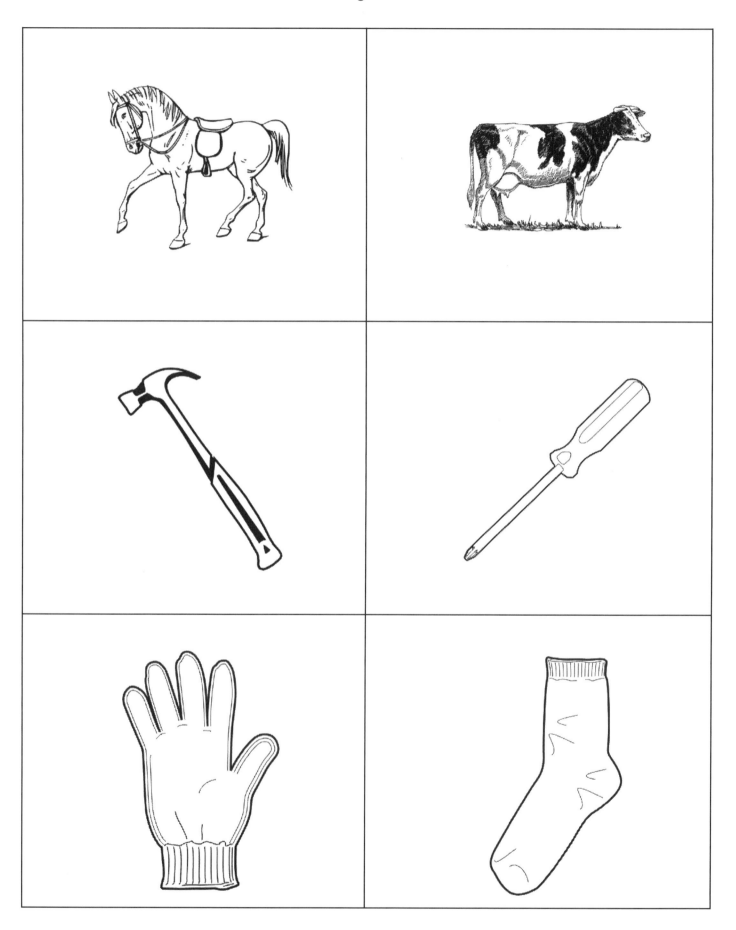

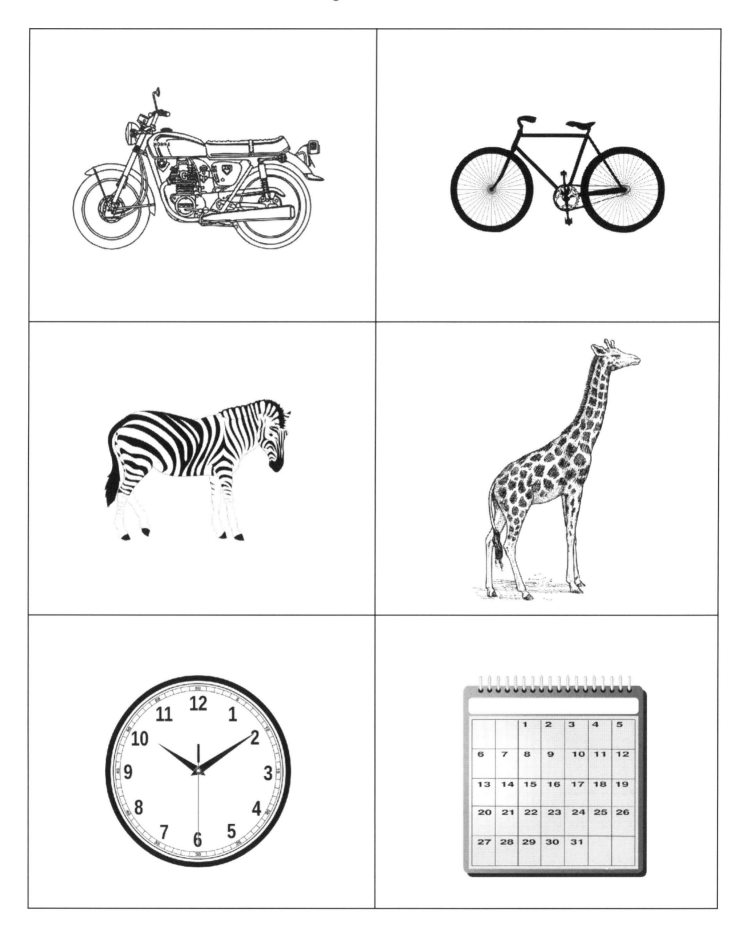

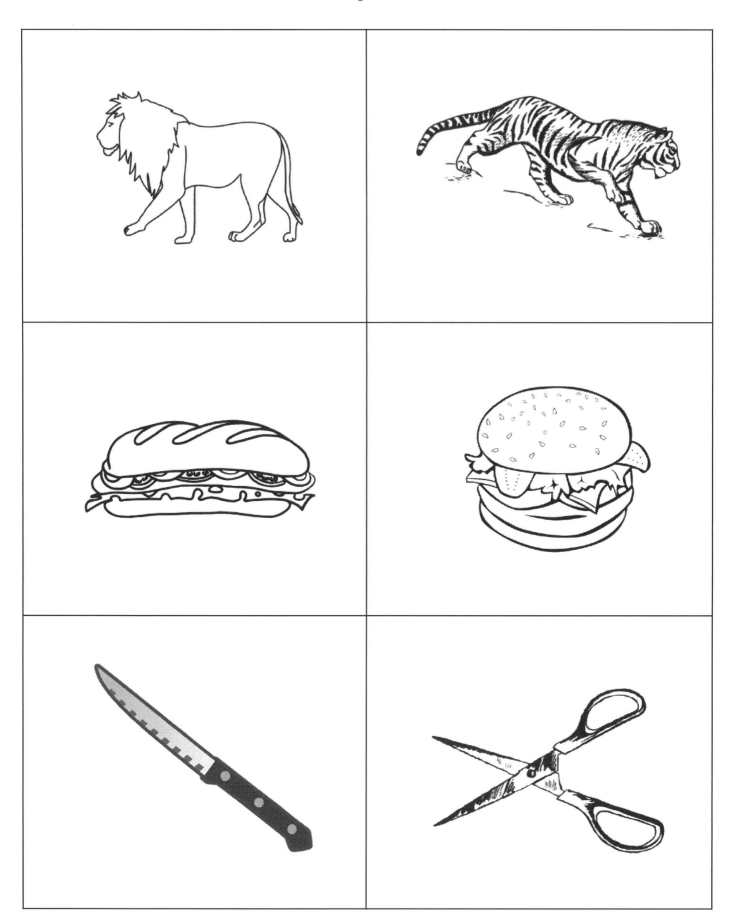

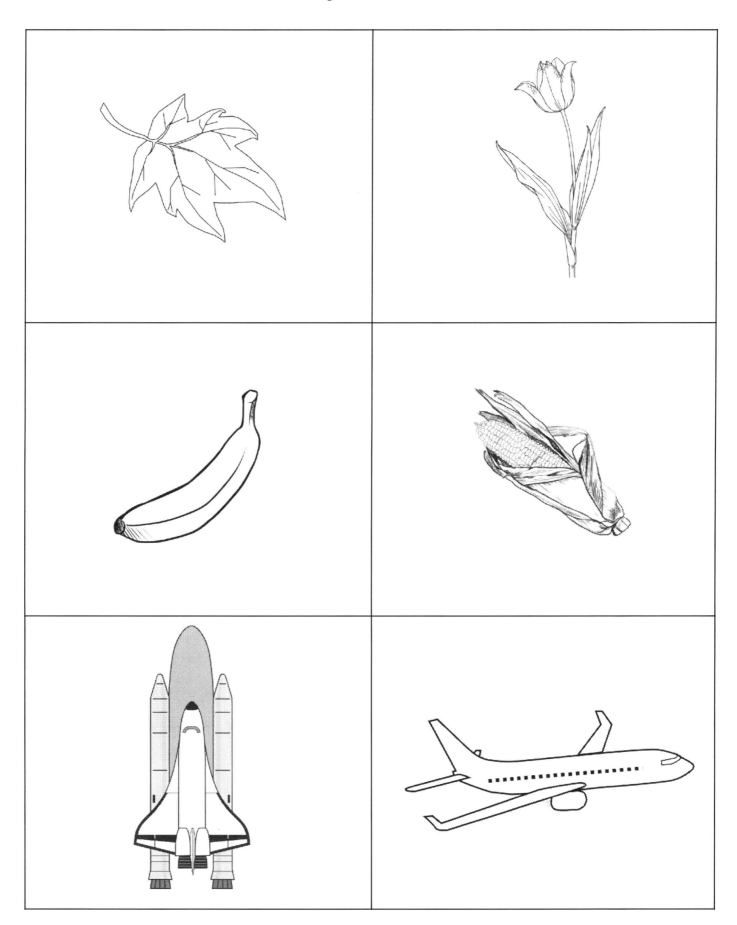

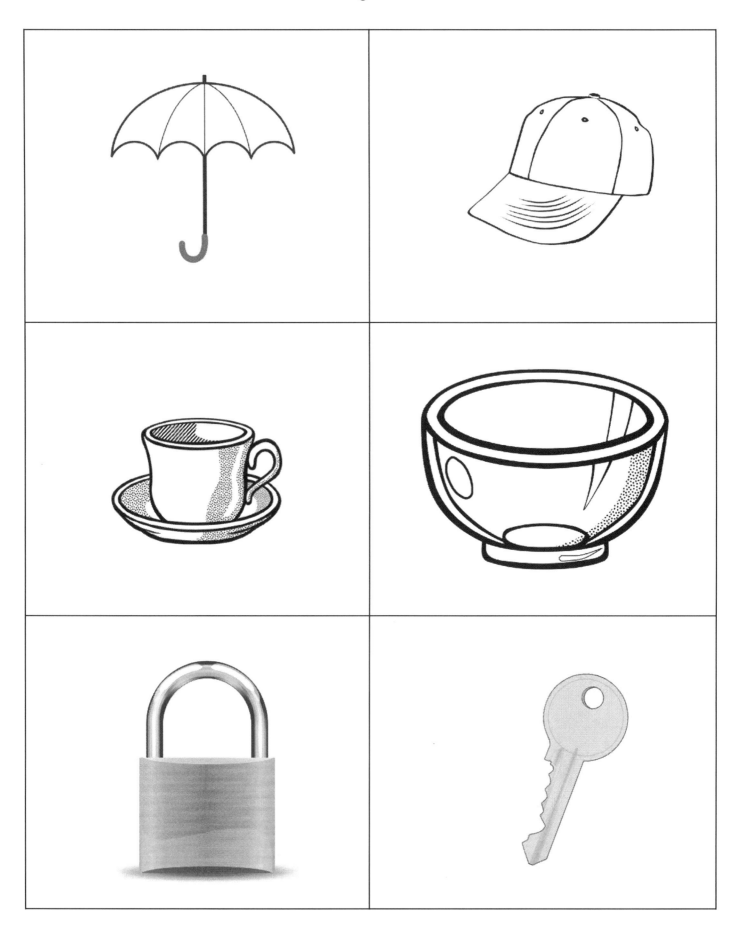

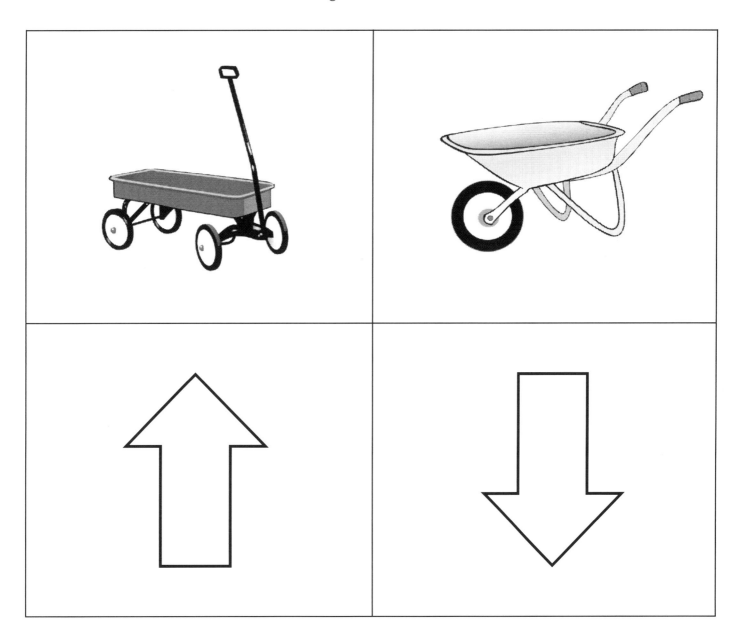

APHASIA

Identify Phrases

Present a pair of phrases to your patient (cover the remaining phrases to avoid confusion). Or write the pair of phrases on a whiteboard. Say one of the phrases aloud. Ask the patient to point to the one you said.

1. Credit Card — Checking Account
2. Rest Area — Restroom
3. Good Luck — Good Bye
4. The end — Table of contents
5. Happy days — Happily ever after
6. Channel guide — Settings menu
7. Changing rooms — Checkout counter
8. Use other door — Push door slowly
9. Unread messages — New voicemail
10. Take as needed — Take daily
11. Building Directory — Main Office
12. Left turn only — Right turn only
13. How are you? — Have a good day!
14. Utility Bill — Phone Bill
15. Local library — Local bank
16. I love you — I like you
17. Salt shaker — Pepper shaker
18. Call ahead — We will call
19. Order Here — Pay Here
20. Pull open — Push open

Phrases & Pictures

Check the phrase that matches the picture.

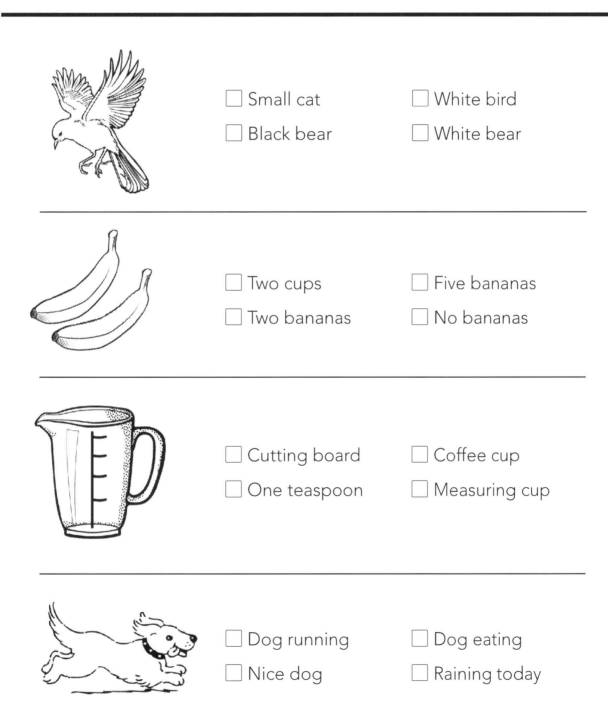

- ☐ Small cat
- ☐ Black bear
- ☐ White bird
- ☐ White bear

- ☐ Two cups
- ☐ Two bananas
- ☐ Five bananas
- ☐ No bananas

- ☐ Cutting board
- ☐ One teaspoon
- ☐ Coffee cup
- ☐ Measuring cup

- ☐ Dog running
- ☐ Nice dog
- ☐ Dog eating
- ☐ Raining today

APHASIA

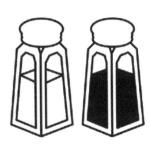

- [ ] Eggs and bacon
- [ ] Salt and pepper
- [ ] Too much salt
- [ ] Black and blue

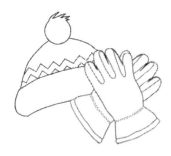

- [ ] Scarf and boots
- [ ] Three gloves
- [ ] Hat and gloves
- [ ] Black hat

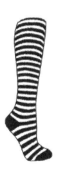

- [ ] Striped sock
- [ ] Short sock
- [ ] Sock and shoe
- [ ] Heavy shoe

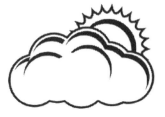

- [ ] Mostly rainy
- [ ] Chance of snow
- [ ] Chance of rain
- [ ] Mostly cloudy

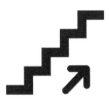

- [ ] Elevator here
- [ ] Go upstairs
- [ ] Go downstairs
- [ ] Office closed

APHASIA

Follow Written Directions

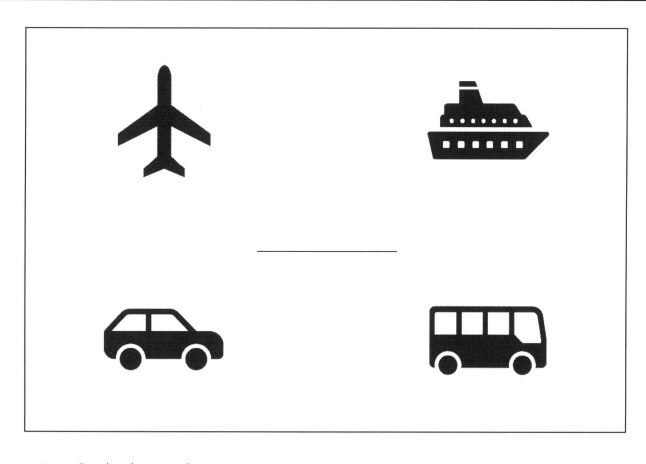

1. Circle the airplane.
2. Place an X on the bus.
3. Underline the ship.
4. Place a checkmark in the middle of the box.
5. Draw a star to the left of the car.

APHASIA

Follow Written Directions

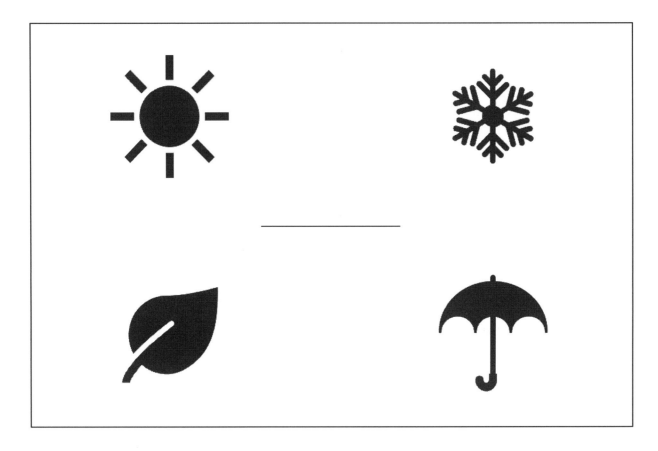

1. Circle the leaf.

2. Draw a star in the middle of the box.

3. Draw a line from the sun to the umbrella.

4. Underline the sun.

5. Place a checkmark to the right of the snowflake.

APHASIA

Follow Written Directions

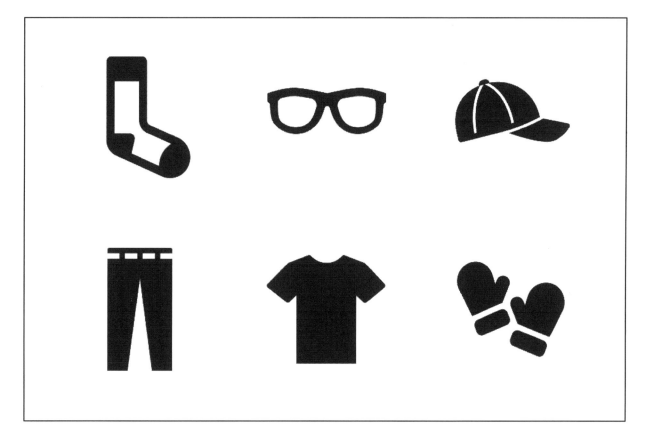

1. Draw a line from the glasses to the mittens.

2. Draw a line from the shirt to the jeans.

3. Draw a circle around the hat.

4. Write your name next to the socks.

5. Underline your name twice.

APHASIA

Follow Written Directions

1. _____

2. _____

3. _____

1. Draw a star on the first line.
2. Draw a checkmark on the last line.
3. Write the word "yes" on the remaining line.
4. Circle the star.
5. Cross out the word on the second line.

> **APHASIA**

Follow Written Directions

---

1. _____

2. _____

3. _____

4. _____

5. _____

1. Write your first name on line 2.
2. Write your birthdate on line 1.
3. Write the name of the city you live in on the last line.
4. Write your age on the line above the city.
5. Draw a star on the remaining line.

APHASIA

Follow Written Directions

Review the directions then complete the steps using the next page.

---

1. Write your first name on the first line.
2. Write your last name on the second line.
3. Write your age on the third line.
4. Write your birthday on the line below your age.
5. Write your initials in the top right square.
6. Place an "X" inside the middle right square.
7. Write the city you live in below your birthday.
8. Write your favorite food on the last line.
9. Write the date on the remaining line.
10. Place one check mark in the remaining square.

APHASIA

Page 2 of 2

1. _____
2. _____
3. _____
4. _____
5. _____
6. _____
7. _____

APHASIA

Identify Sentences

Present a pair of sentences to your patient (cover the remaining sentences to avoid confusion). Or write the pair of sentences on a whiteboard. Say one of the sentences aloud. Ask the patient to point to the one you said.

1. Good to see you! — It was good seeing you!
2. Thank you for your payment. — Please enclose your payment.
3. Your appointment is at noon. — Breakfast is served until noon.
4. We open again on Monday. — We close early on Sunday.
5. Side effects include dizziness. — You may experience side effects.
6. Take one pill with water. — Take on an empty stomach.
7. Do your exercises twice a day. — Exercise at least two times daily.
8. She is on leave until April. — She is retiring in April.
9. We look forward to your call. — Please call at your earliest convenience.
10. Place your hands on 10 and 2. — Please arrive between 10 and 2.
11. Do you know the way home? — Do you know the way back?
12. What a terrible surprise. — What a terrific surprise.
13. I hope to arrive early. — An early arrival is what I hope for.
14. Did you not go to the doctor? — You did not go to the doctor?
15. The car hit the raccoon. — The raccoon was hit by the car.

APHASIA

Paragraphs

Read each paragraph aloud to your patient then ask the related questions.

1. Sara had a dinner party at 7 pm. She wanted to do some chores before the guests arrived, but cooking took longer than expected. The dinner was delicious.
    - When was Sara's dinner party?
    - Why didn't she do some chores?
    - How did the food turn out?

2. Karindy went to the store to buy cough syrup. However, the store only had cough drops and herbal tea. She bought both, and her cough was gone by the next day.
    - Why did Karindy go to the store?
    - What did she buy at the store?
    - Did her cough get better?

3. Miss Whitson took her dogs out for a walk. Their normal route was blocked by construction, but the new route she chose was beautiful. They walked over two miles.
    - Who did Miss Whitson walk with?
    - Why didn't she take her normal route?
    - How far did they walk?

APHASIA

4. Christy had always wanted to learn how to play the guitar, so she found a tutor online. She was a natural and learned quickly. Now, she plays at bars on open mic nights. The audiences love her sets.
   - What is the woman's name?
   - What did she always want to learn?
   - Where does she perform?

5. Falah was excited for a family trip to California. They planned to visit Disneyland, Hollywood, and the beach. Needing a car large enough to fit all of her siblings, she rented a minivan. Falah hoped they would have enough time to visit the zoo.
   - Where was Falah going?
   - What kind of vehicle did she rent?
   - Where else did Falah hope to go?

6. Mr. McHenry loved going to the theatre with his wife, especially to watch musicals. The only problem was that his wife often fell asleep during the show. This upset him. He asked his wife what would help her to stay awake. The next time they visited the theater, he gave her several pieces of gum. She stayed awake the entire show!
   - What types of shows did Mr. McHenry like the most?
   - Why was he upset with his wife?
   - What did he give his wife at the next show?

APHASIA

7. Kim was training for a 5K foot race with her friends. She was nervous because she hadn't raced since her surgery, two years earlier. She asked her neighbor, a marathon runner, for advice. He suggested that she run at least four times a week, stretch before and after each run, and invest in good running shoes. Kim followed her neighbor's advice and was glad she did. She felt great during the race!
   - What was Kim training for?
   - What happened to her two years earlier?
   - What did Kim's neighbor suggest she do to prepare for the race?

8. JaToya was in the last term of fashion design school. Her final project was to design a runway collection featuring 12 of her original designs. She had designed dresses, skirts, and hats for her six models, but she was struggling to come up with a show-stopper piece. One day, she had a flash of inspiration when a hummingbird flew by her window. JaToya designed a jacket embroidered with emerald green, red, and purple. Her collection was a hit!
   - What type of school did JaToya attend?
   - How many designs did she need to create?
   - What inspired her show-stopper piece?
   - What was her show-stopper piece?

9. Nico moved to Alaska over the summer to take his very first job as a high school counselor. That summer, he enjoyed hiking, fishing, and kayaking. Once school started, despite the long hours, Nico loved working with his students. It wasn't until winter that he began to doubt his move to Alaska: The sun set before 4 pm and he'd once woken to find a bear on his back porch. His students suggested that he put up more lamps to brighten his house and that he clean his porch thoroughly to avoid attracting bears. The suggestions worked! But Nico was still relieved when summer arrived.
    - Where did Nico move to?
    - What was his new job?
    - Why did he end up doubting his move to Alaska?

APHASIA

10. Blake was running late for his son's class play. He meant to leave work 30 minutes early but ended up staying late to help a coworker who was having computer trouble. After fixing the issue, Blake rushed home. He picked up the three dozen cupcakes he and his son Daniel had baked the night before, then drove to the school. He arrived just as the performance began. The play was about George Washington's childhood and Daniel was the cherry tree. The entire audience laughed when he shouted, "TIMBER!" and toppled over. Daniel noticed him in the audience, and Blake gave his son a huge, proud smile.
    - What is the father's name?
    - Why was he late?
    - What did he pick up at home?
    - What part did Daniel play?

APHASIA

11. Yadai was born in South Korea to American parents. Both of her parents worked for the U.S. government, and they moved every few years. Although Yadai lived all around the world, she always felt a special connection to South Korea. After graduating from college, Yadai took a full-time job in Seoul. Through language classes and with the help of patient coworkers, she began to learn Korean. One of her coworkers was a Korean native named Jin, and they became fast friends. No one was surprised when, a year later, Yadai and Jin announced their engagement. Their wedding will be an outdoor ceremony in the fall. Yadai is now fluent in Korean, although Jin still corrects her conjugations every now and then.
    - Where was Yadai born?
    - Who did her parents work for?
    - In what city did Yadai get her full-time job?
    - When is she getting married?
    - What is her fiancé's name?

Reading

Read the paragraph aloud then summarize what you read.

---

1. Washington state is known for being a rainy place. This is not unfounded, as some of its cities have over 140 rainy days per year. Washington rain, however, is usually a light drizzle. When measuring total inches of rain per year, Washington is only the 29th rainiest state. The frequency of rainy days in the western part of the state makes it a green, vibrant place most of the year. Locals know to invest to good waterproof jackets.

2. Black Friday is a huge shopping day for Americans. It takes place on the Friday after Thanksgiving and is considered the start of the holiday shopping season. The term "Black Friday" was coined in the 1960s and referred to the increased holiday traffic on that day. For years, stores opened at 6 am on Black Friday. However, some big-box retailers now open at 4 am, midnight, or even on Thanksgiving day.

3. Osaka, pronounced "OH-saw-ka," is the second largest city in Japan. It is also one of the largest cities in the world, with a population of over 20 million people. Osaka is considered Japan's economic center. It is home to electronics giants Panasonic, Sharp, and Sanyo. Osaka is also one of the most expensive cities in the world to live in—more expensive even than New York City or Los Angeles.

4. Siberians cats are a breed of domestic cats that originated in Siberia. They are the national cat breed of Russia. Siberian cats have developed thick, soft fur that protects them from harsh winters. Their fur also produces less allergens than most other cat breeds, leading some to claim that they are hypoallergenic. While not completely hypoallergenic, many with cat allergies say that they are not allergic to these pets.

APHASIA

5. A stroke occurs after blood flow to the brain becomes interrupted. They are sometimes called "brain attacks" in reference to heart attacks (which occur after blood flow to your heart is interrupted). Risk factors for stroke include high blood pressure, diabetes, smoking, and advanced age. The occurrence of strokes increases on Christmas and New Year's Day. This is because the holidays can be a stressful time and people consume more alcohol and fatty foods. To reduce your risk for stroke, doctors recommend eating right, exercising, reducing stress, and taking your medications.

6. The film "Gone with the Wind" was released in 1939. It is set during the reconstruction era following the American Civil War. It was a huge hit upon its release with both critics and audiences. Vivien Leigh's performance as Scarlett O'Hara was particularly praised. The film won 10 Academy Awards, including Best Picture, Best Director, Best Actress, and Best Supporting Actress. For decades, it was the highest grossing film of all time. Even today, when adjusted for inflation, it remains the highest grossing film of all time, making over $3 billion worldwide.

7. The digits 0 to 9 are Arabic numerals. They are the most common way to represent numbers. Arabic numerals were developed around the year 700 AD in India before spreading to the Middle East and North Africa. Around 1200 AD, Leonardo Fibonacci helped introduce the numerals to Europe. The numerals became more widely known throughout Europe thanks to the invention of the printing press. By the 1400s, Arabic numbers were inscribed into churches to mark when they were constructed. These days, computer code uses Arabic numerals.

8. Daylight saving time was first proposed in 1895. It was officially established in the U.S. in 1918, in the same law that enacted time zones across the country. Daylight saving time was repealed just a year later but then re-established during World War II. After the war, states varied on enforcement of daylight saving. In 1966, the Time Uniform Act standardized when daylight saving time would begin and end.

APHASIA

Everyday Reading

Review the everyday reading material on the next page then answer the questions.

---

1. Where is this weather forecast for?
   _____

2. What day is it?
   _____

3. What days will it be showering?
   _____

4. What day will it be partly sunny?
   _____

5. What time is it?
   _____

APHASIA

Page 2 of 2

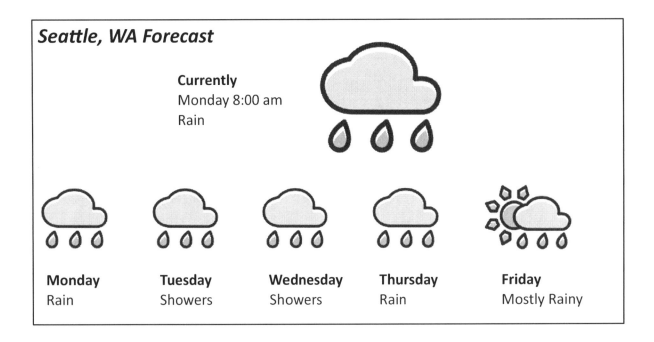

APHASIA

Everyday Reading

Review the everyday reading material on the next page then answer the questions.

---

1. What is this Table of Contents for?
   _____

2. What page is "Definitions" on?
   _____

3. What page is "Waiver" on?
   _____

4. Does "Contacts" come before "FAQs"?
   _____

5. What types of Health benefits are available?
   _____

Member Benefits Information Packet for the 2022-2023 Year

Introduction	1
Definitions	3
Health Benefits	7
PPO	10
HMO	15
Vision	19
Dental	22
Forms	24
Waiver	28
FAQs	30
Contacts	34

APHASIA

Everyday Reading

Review the everyday reading material on the next page then answer the questions.

---

1. Who wrote this card?
   _____

2. Who received this card?
   _____

3. What happened to her?
   _____

4. When was this card written?
   _____

5. What food was mentioned?
   _____

APHASIA

Page 2 of 2

12/10/2021

Satomi—

Get Better Soon!

I hope your surgery went well. We will come by to visit once you're back on your feet. I'll bring my famous cornbread, and we'll call it a party!

Love,
Yoko & Jordan

| APHASIA |

Everyday Reading

Review the everyday reading material on the next page then answer the questions.

1. What is the name of the grocery store?
   _____

2. How long are these deals good for?
   _____

3. How much is salmon?
   _____

4. Is salt cheaper than a lemon?
   _____

5. What is the cheapest meat per pound?
   _____

Bargain Market
Weekly Deals

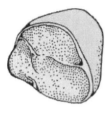
Ham $5.99 lb

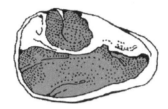
Sirloin Steaks $7.99 lb

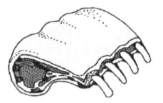
Pork Ribs $4.99 lb

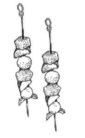
Pork Kabobs $4 ea

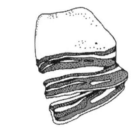
Farm Cut Bacon $2.99 lb

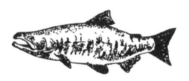
Atlantic Salmon $9.99 lb

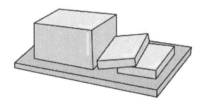
Local Butter $4.39

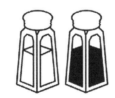
Salt or Pepper $1.29

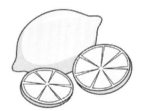
Large Lemons $0.69

Everyday Reading

Review the everyday reading material on the next page then answer the questions.

1. What is the name of this restaurant?

2. Can you buy a cheeseburger at this restaurant?

3. Can you buy a bacon cheeseburger at this restaurant?

4. What can you add to the fries?

5. What type of sauce can you buy?

6. What's the most expensive add-on on the menu?

7. What are the cheapest add-ons?

8. Is a drink more expensive than adding gravy and cheese curds?

ORI'S BURGERS

BURGER $6.00

+ CHEDDAR CHEESE $1.00

+BACON $2.00

+ SPECIAL SAUCE $1.00

FRIES $5.00

+ SPECIAL SAUCE $1.00

+ GRAVY AND CHEESE CURDS $4.00

DRINKS $2.50

Everyday Reading

Review the everyday reading material on the next page then answer the questions.

---

1. What is the name of this restaurant?
   _____

2. How much does coffee cost?
   _____

3. How much does a fruit cup cost?
   _____

4. What item(s) cost $4.50?
   _____

5. What is the cheapest item?
   _____

Dominic's Café

DRINKS
Coffee $2.50
Tea $2.00
Latte $4.00
Cappuccino $4.00
Mocha $4.50
Hot Chocolate $3.50

SNACKS
Biscotti $2.50
Bagel $3.50
Muffin $3.00
Scone $3.50
Cake Slice $4.50
Fruit Cup $4.00

APHASIA

Everyday Reading

Review the everyday reading material on the next page then answer the questions.

1. What is the name of this restaurant?
   _____

2. How many types of cheese can you buy here?
   _____

3. What other types of food can you buy here?
   _____

4. How many types of spreads can you buy here?
   _____

5. How much does one item cost?
   _____

6. How much do five items cost?
   _____

7. Can you buy more than six items here?
   _____

8. How much would gouda, multigrain crackers, and dark chocolate cost (three items)?
   _____

Ye Olde Cheese Shoppe

CHEESE: Aged Cheddar, Brie, Muenster, Gorgonzola, Gouda

CRACKERS: Multigrain, Cracked Pepper, Rosemary, Cheese

MEAT: Summer Sausage, Prosciutto, Hard Salami, Turkey Sausage

SPREADS: Orange Marmalade, Blackberry Preserves, Apple Butter

SWEETS: Hard Candy, Dark Chocolate, Peppermint, Licorice

$5 One item, $9 Two items, $14 Three items, $18 Four items, $22 Five items, $25 Six items, plus $3 Each item after six items

| APHASIA | *Page 1 of 2* |

Everyday Reading

Review the everyday reading material on the next page then answer the questions.

---

1. Who is the passenger?
   _____

2. What is his seat number?
   _____

3. What is his boarding zone?
   _____

4. Where is he going?
   _____

5. What is his flight number?
   _____

6. What airlines is he flying?
   _____

7. What date is he flying?
   _____

8. When is his departure time?
   _____

APHASIA

Page 2 of 2

REGRETTABLE AIRLINES

FLIGHT
RA 1313

DESTINATION
SEA TO HEL

PASSENGER
TURNIP, NED

PASSENGER
TURNIP, NED

SEAT
35G

GATE
F13

DEPARTURE
12:01 AM 10 APR 2022

BOARDING ZONE
C4

TRACKING
233 982 2341

DATA
00 41 N

SEATING CLASS
ECONOMY MINUS

APHASIA

Everyday Reading

Review the everyday reading material on the next page then answer the questions.

---

1. How many servings are there per each container?
   _____

2. What is the serving size?
   _____

3. How many grams of protein are there per serving?
   _____

4. How many grams of sugar are there per serving?
   _____

5. Is there any saturated fat?
   _____

APHASIA

Texas-Sized CHEESE BALLS

Nutrition Facts

64 servings per container

Serving size   2 cheese balls

Amount per serving

Calories 545

% Daily Value*

Total Fat 8g	10%
Saturated Fat 2g	7%
Trans Fat 0g	
Cholesterol <5mg	1%
Sodium 250mg	11%
Total Carbohydrate 17g	7%
Dietary Fiber 1g	4%
Total Sugars 1g	
Includes 0g Added Sugars	0%
Protein 5g	8%

Not a significant source of vitamin D, calcium, iron, and potassium.

*The % Daily Value (DV) tells you how much a nutrient in a serving of food contributes to a daily diet. 2,000 calories a day is used for general nutrition advice.

APHASIA

Everyday Reading

Review the everyday reading material on the next page then answer the questions.

---

1. Who is this prescription for?
   _____

2. Who is the prescribing doctor?
   _____

3. What pharmacy filled this prescription?
   _____

4. Where is the pharmacy located?
   _____

5. When was the prescription filled?
   _____

6. Are there any remaining refills?
   _____

7. How many tablets are in the prescription bottle?
   _____

8. What is the dosage of each tablet?
   _____

APHASIA

MAIN STREET PHARMACY RX#0001719

SPORK, WANDA
DOB: 05/20/65

CHILLIZIDE 500MG TABLET
TAKE ONE TABLET ONCE DAILY.

PRESCRIBED BY: FREEZE, A.

QTY: 30   DATE FILLED: 10/10/2022
2 REFILLS REMAIN   DISCARD BY: 10/10/2023

400 MAIN STREET #3
LOGJAM, WA 98001   398-398-4400

| APHASIA | *Page 1 of 2* |

Everyday Reading

Review the everyday reading material on the next page then answer the questions.

---

1. Who is this prescription for?
   _____

2. Who was the prescribing doctor?
   _____

3. What pharmacy filled this prescription?
   _____

4. What does the tablet look like?
   _____

5. When was the prescription created?
   _____

6. Are there any remaining refills?
   _____

7. How many tablets are in the prescription bottle?
   _____

8. What type of tablet is it?
   _____

APHASIA

DRUGS 'R US   404-800-8080
5454 Science St.
Pumpkins, CA 91301

RX#00072001   Date filled 08/01/2021
Original RX 08/01/2021

BOYD, BENJAMIN
6001 Morning Road
Pumpkins, CA 91301

VITAMIN TABLET 1,000 MG
WHITE OVAL 110

TAKE ONE (1) TABLET TWICE DAILY FOR TWO WEEKS.
THEN ONE (1) TABLET ONCE DAILY.

Px: Janet Sheep, M.D.   MFR: Generic Vitamin Co.
404-505-2200

QTY: 45
REFILL 5 TIMES UNTIL 07/31/2022   DISCARD AFTER 08/01/2022

APHASIA

Everyday Reading

Review the everyday reading material on the next page then answer the questions.

---

1. What store is this receipt for?
   _____

2. Who was the cashier?
   _____

3. What was the subtotal?
   _____

4. How much was the ketchup?
   _____

5. What type of payment was used?
   _____

APHASIA

Thank you for shopping at
Ready Mart

9055 Treeline Lane
Springfield, MO 46460

02/14/2022   08:45 AM
Term ID: ****004
Cashier: Brad

Item Count: 8
==================================
1 BOTTLED WATER 24 CT $5.99
1 BUNS HOT DOG 8 CT $3.69
1 ALL BEEF HOT DOG $5.99
1 SAUERKRAUT 16 OZ $3.99
1 KETCHUP 12 OZ $2.19
1 MUSTARD 8 OZ $1.89
1 MARSHMALLOW 11.5 OZ $2.39
1 BEER 6 CT $6.99
==================================
SUBTOTAL $33.12
SALES TAX $0.00
LIQUOR TAX $0.69
GRAND TOTAL $33.81

CREDIT SALE
ACCT #: ************VISA 0411
REF #: 245891
AUTH CODE: 182223

APHASIA

Everyday Reading

Review the everyday reading material on the next page then answer the questions.

1. What month was this statement for?
   _____

2. Whose statement is this?
   _____

3. What is the ending balance?
   _____

4. What was the beginning balance?
   _____

5. What are the last four digits of the account number?
   _____

6. What bank is this?
   _____

7. Where was $17.14 spent?
   _____

City Credit Union   **Statement Ending 04/30/2022**

RETURN SERVICE REQUESTED

Anita Flores
732 Wagon Wheel Ct.
Springfield, MO 63434

CITY CREDIT UNION CHECKING-XXXXX0498

Primary Checking
Account Summary

Date	Description	Amount
04/01/2022	Beginning Balance	$987.56
	3 Credits This Period	$3,300.50
	20 Debits This Period	
04/30/2022	Ending Balance	$1,611.04

Account Activity

Post Date	Description	Debits	Credits	Balance
04/01/2022	Check #119	$800.00		$187.56
04/01/2022	DIRECT DEP		$1,600.00	$1787.56
04/04/2022	Jackie's Diner	$37.67		$1749.89
04/04/2022	Sweet Treats	$14.99		$1734.90
04/06/2022	City of Springfield	$234.00		$1500.90
04/08/2022	Buylots.com	$89.54		$1411.36
04/09/2022	ATM DEPOSIT		$100.00	$1511.36
04/12/2022	Gas N Go	$35.23		$1476.13
04/12/2022	Burger Burger	$17.14		$1458.99
04/15/2022	DIRECT DEP		$1600.50	$3059.49
04/16/2022	Furniture Mart	$886.86		$2172.63

Everyday Reading

Review the everyday reading material on the next page then answer the questions.

1. What award was given?
   _____

2. Who won the award?
   _____

3. What does the winner receive with the award?
   _____

4. How many people were nominated?
   _____

5. Who wrote this letter?
   _____

Abigail Fresh
123 Journey Lane
Lake Jackson, TX 77001

July 5, 2021

Dear Mrs. Fresh,

    You were nominated by your associates for our annual "Clinician of the Year" award. This year, we received over 7,000 nominations nationwide. We are pleased to inform you that our committee has selected you as Clinician of the Year for 2021!

    Our committee was blown away by your commitment to patients, your use of humor to improve clinical outcomes, and your unbiased compassion for people of all backgrounds.

    The Clinician of the Year is awarded a $10,000 grant, an all-expense-paid trip to the awards ceremony in Austin, and exclusive bragging rights for the entire year.

    We look forward to meeting you in person and will contact you shortly to solidify travel plans.

    Thank you for all that you do and congratulations!

Jeong-Hee Brewster
Chair, Clinician of the Year Association

APHASIA

Picture Description

Presenting one photo at a time, ask the patient to describe each image in as much detail as possible.

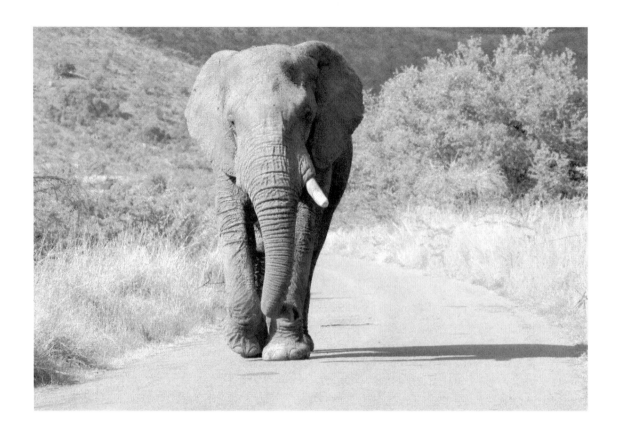

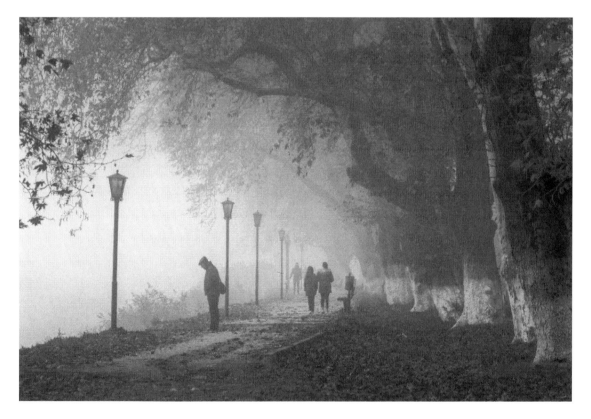

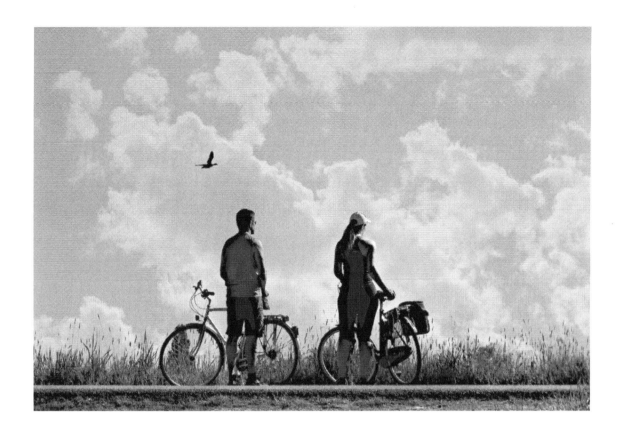
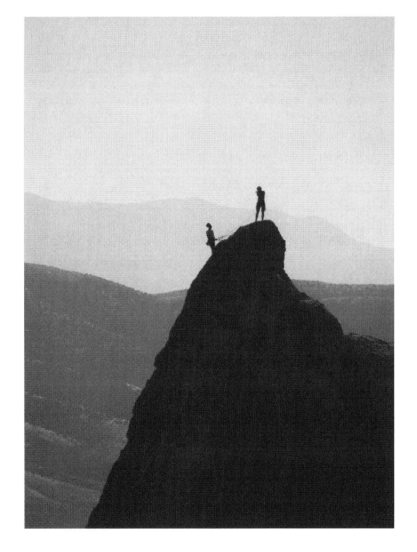

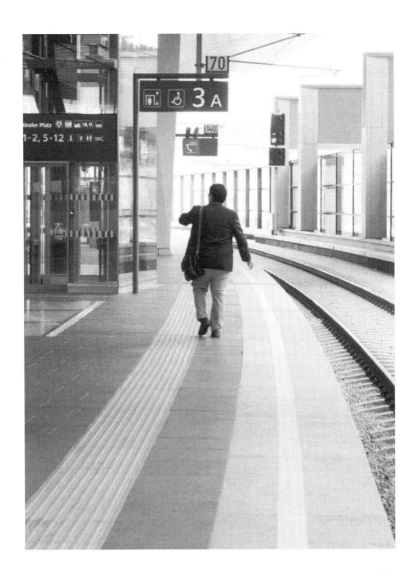

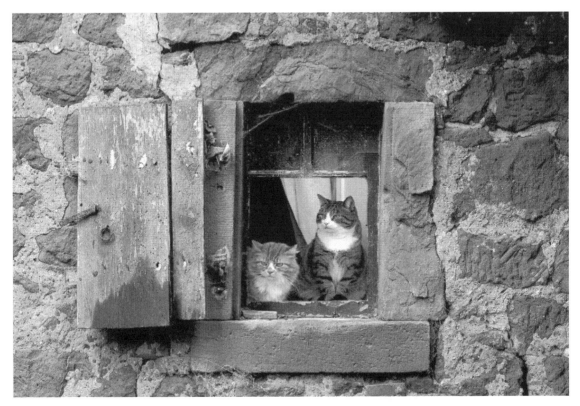

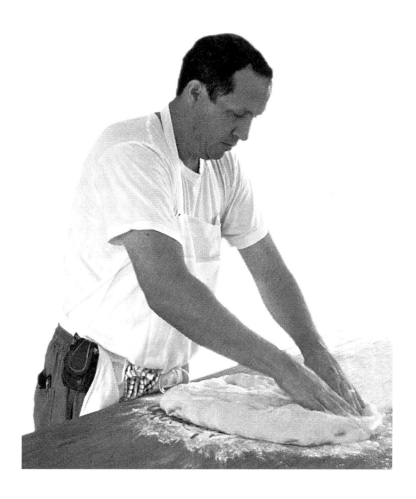

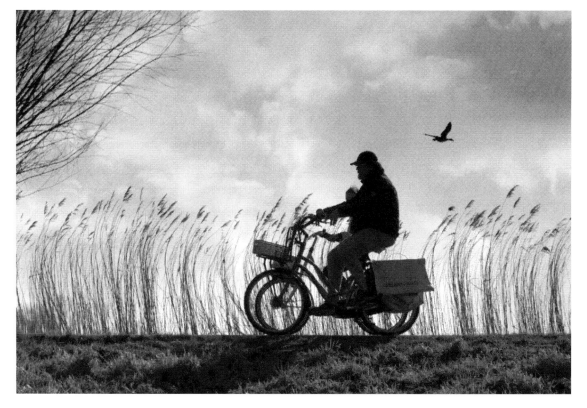

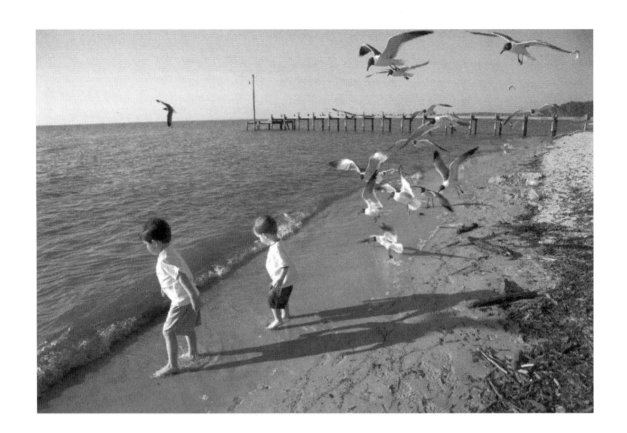

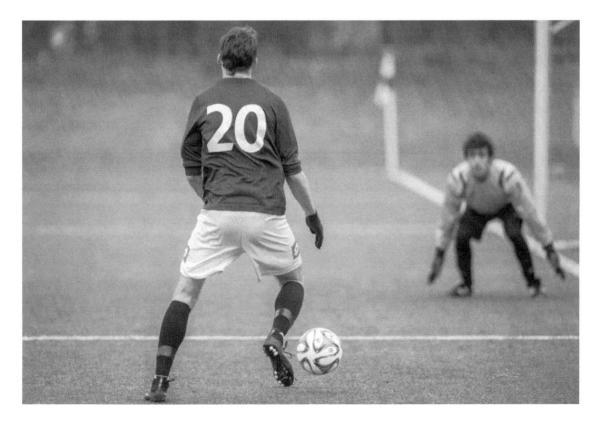

MOTOR SPEECH

Motor speech disorders involve muscle weakness or difficulty coordinating the muscles used for speech. They include acquired apraxia of speech and dysarthria. The goal of motor speech treatment is to increase the effectiveness and naturalness of communication by improving respiration, phonation, articulation, resonance, and/or prosody. For patients with progressive diseases, maintaining function is the goal of treatment. Choose motor speech goals and techniques based on the patient's previous and current levels of functioning, nature of the disease/disability (e.g., acute or progressive), amount of support available, motivation, and other relevant factors.

Motor speech treatment includes:
- Restorative treatment (e.g. increasing muscle strength)
- Compensatory approaches (e.g. using clear speech strategies)
- AAC and other modalities
- Identifying any needed accommodations, including environmental modifications

MOTOR SPEECH

Therapist Instructions

EVALUATIONS. Motor speech evaluations consist of a case history, oral mechanism examination, connected speech and reading sample, assessment of diadochokinetic rate, repetition of words and phrases, naming, picture description, and tests for limb and oral apraxia.
- Formal evaluations include the *Word Intelligibility Test* and *Assessment of Intelligibility in Dysarthric Speech*.

DAY ONE OF TREATMENT. Provide the following handouts, as needed.
- Homework Log, Monthly Calendar, Motor Speech Impairments, Intelligibility Tips, Listener Tips, Clear Speech Strategies, Inspiratory Checking, Diaphragmatic Breathing, Alphabet Board
- Highlight key points on the handouts, then review with your patients. Ask questions to make sure they understand the content. Answer any questions they may have.

FOR THERAPIST EYES ONLY. Pages marked with a gray background or header are resources for therapists. Some caregivers and patients may benefit from having a copy.
- Motor Learning, Sound Production Treatment, Minimal Pairs, Phone Calls, Conversation, Interview, Monologues

STRATEGIES. Select 2-3 of the most pertinent strategies for each patient. Review the selected strategies, provide a model, then ask for return demonstrations. Have these handouts available each session and refer to them often.
- Intelligibility Tips, Clear Speech Strategies, Inspiratory Checking, Diaphragmatic Breathing, Breath Control, Building Up Breath Control, Alphabet Board

PRONUNCIATIONS. Pronunciations are based on a General American English dialect. If needed, modify the Heteronyms (page 461) and Phonemic Lists (page 464) to accommodate for your patient's accent.

MOTOR SPEECH

RESPIRATION. Use Intelligibility Tips, Listener Tips, Inspiratory Checking, Diaphragmatic Breathing, Breath Control, and Building Up Breath Control for difficulty coordinating respiration for speech.
- Print out reading material and add slash marks between words to denote a new breath group. Where you add the slash mark will depend on each patient's skill level.
- See the Voice & Resonance chapter (page 531) for more information about muscle strength training.

ARTICULATION. Use Intelligibility Tips, Listener Tips, Clear Speech Strategies, Building Up Breath Control, Alphabet Board, Phones Calls, Conversation, Interview, Monologues, and Phonemic Lists to treat articulation difficulties.

PROSODY. Use the Building Up Breath Control, Sentence Stress, and Heteronyms worksheets to treat prosody difficulties.

PHONATION. Use the speech breathing illustration (page 451) to treat phonation difficulties. See the Voice & Resonance chapter for more information about *LSVT LOUD®*, amplification, and other treatments.

RESONANCE. See the Voice & Resonance chapter (pages 537–539) for resources.

READING MATERIAL. Additional reading material can be found in the Aphasia, Memory, and Visual Neglect chapters.
- Prompt your patients to ask themselves, "How did my talking sound?" This teaches them to monitor their own speech.

CRANIOFACIAL & ENT REFERRALS. Some patients with motor speech disorders may benefit from seeing craniofacial specialists or otolaryngologists (ENT doctors). These professionals can identify and manage structural issues in the head and neck and innervation issues. Some patients may need procedures prior to receiving speech therapy (e.g., palatal lift prosthesis or nasal obturator).

MOTOR SPEECH

Contents

Motor Learning	438
Sound Production Treatment	440
Minimal Pairs	442
Motor Speech Impairments	443
Intelligibility Tips	444
Listener Tips	445
Clear Speech Strategies	446
Inspiratory Checking	447
Diaphragmatic Breathing	448
Diaphragm Illustration	449
Breath Control	450
Building Up Breath Control	452
Alphabet Board *(for motor speech)*	453
Phone Calls	454
Conversation	455
Interview	456
Monologues	457
Sentence Stress	458
Heteronyms	461

PHONEMIC LISTS

/p/	465
/b/	468
/m/	471
/w/	474
/f/	477

MOTOR SPEECH

/v/	480
"th"	483
/d/	486
/t/	489
/n/	492
/s/	495
/z/	498
/ɹ/	501
/l/	504
/k/	507
/g/	510
/ʃ/	513
/tʃ/	516
/dʒ/	519
/ʒ/ medial and final	522
/j/	523
/h/	526

SEE ALSO

Giving Directions	355
Differences Between Words	356
Definitions	357
Conversations	358
Reading	395
Alphabet Board	569

Motor Learning

When treating apraxia, dysarthria, and other motor speech disorders, a common goal is to facilitate motor learning; you are helping the patient learn new movements. Motor learning results in a permanent change to how the patient moves. It comes from lots of practice in many different contexts. The principles of motor learning are described below (Bislick et al., 2012).

PRE-PRACTICE. Make sure that patients are: 1) motivated, 2) understand expectations (i.e. what a "correct" answer is and why), and 3) are stimulable for the treatment you chose.

USE A LARGE NUMBER OF TRIALS. Aim for at least 50 repetitions per target.

USE DISTRIBUTED PRACTICE. Distributed practice is having a given number of trials or sessions over a longer period of time (Maas et al., 2008). For example, your patient has 20 sessions of therapy. With distributed practice, you schedule 2 sessions per week for 10 weeks.
- In contrast, an example of a massed practice schedule is 4 sessions per week for 5 weeks. Massed practice can be effective and is used in some treatments (e.g. LSVT LOUD).

USE VARIABLE PRACTICE. Practice different targets in different ways. For example, the patient produces several different phonemes in different word positions.
- In the early stages of treatment, some patients may need to practice the same target in the same way (e.g. they first produce a specific phoneme in word-initial position).

USE RANDOM PRACTICE. Practice different targets in random order. For example, the patient targets two phonemes in random order throughout an entire session.
- In the early stages of treatment or with a severe impairment, patients may need to practice each target individually (e.g. they produce one target phoneme for the first half of the session then another target phoneme for the second half).

MOTOR SPEECH

USE COMPLEX PRACTICE. "Complex" refers to the whole movement; the sum of all its parts. Learning a complex movement improves motor learning of both the complex and simple movements. For example, saying a multisyllabic word is a complex movement while saying an individual phoneme in that word is a simple movement.
- Some patients may benefit from practicing individual parts of the task first.

PROVIDE FEEDBACK. Give patients feedback about how they performed. Feedback may be general ("Not quite") or specific ("Bring your lips closer together for that sound"). You can also provide biofeedback.

PROVIDE REDUCED FEEDBACK. Reduced feedback (e.g. giving feedback after 50% or 20% of trials) can help patients self-monitor, instead of being dependent on therapist feedback. This improves motor learning.
- Given reduced feedback, patients with apraxia of speech and dysarthria have higher retention of learning than those given frequent feedback. Their task performance may be low during the session, but retention (or motor learning) is higher (Maas et al., 2008).
- In the early stages of treatment, patients may benefit from frequent feedback to acquire the new movement.

PROVIDE DELAYED FEEDBACK. Wait 5 seconds after the trial before giving feedback. This allows the patient enough time to evaluate their own performance first.
- That said, immediate feedback can be helpful for some with apraxia of speech.

MOTOR SPEECH

Sound Production Treatment for Apraxia

This approach can improve a patient's motor programming abilities *(Wambaugh & Mauszycki, 2010)*.

Prepare a set of 30 or more minimal pairs that focus on the patient's errors (see page 442).

Progress to the next step only if the patient is **incorrect**. At the first correct answer, ask for 5 repetitions: Provide feedback for accuracy ~3 of the 5 repetitions to enhance motor learning.

STEP 1:
MODEL the target word. Ask for repetition.

CORRECT:
Ask for 5 more repetitions.
Move to a new word on Step 1.

INCORRECT:
Provide feedback. Say, "Let's try a different word."
Model the **minimal pair** word. Ask for repetition.

CORRECT:
Provide feedback.
Say, "Let's go back to the other word."
Advance to STEP 2.

INCORRECT:
Provide feedback. Use the **minimal pair** word and say, **"Watch me, listen to me, say it with me."** Repeat up to 3 times.

CORRECT:
Provide feedback.
Advance to STEP 2.

INCORRECT:
Provide feedback.
Advance to STEP 2.

MOTOR SPEECH

STEP 2:
WRITE down the target sound. Model the TARGET WORD. Ask for repetition.

For example, the word is "ten." The target sound is the /t/, so write down the letter "t."

CORRECT: Ask for 5 more repetitions. Move to a new word on Step 1.	INCORRECT: **Advance to STEP 3.**

STEP 3:
Continue using the target word.
Say, "Watch me, listen to me, say it with me." Repeat up to 3 times.

CORRECT. Ask for 5 more repetitions. Move to a new word on Step 1.	INCORRECT: **Advance to STEP 4.**

STEP 4:
Provide ARTICULATORY PLACEMENT cues. Say, "Watch me, listen to me, say it with me."

CORRECT. Ask for 5 more repetitions. Move to a new word on Step 1.	INCORRECT: **Move to a new word on Step 1.**

MOTOR SPEECH

Minimal Pairs

Example minimal pairs for use with Sound Production Treatment.

1. Ten/Hen
2. Name/Lame
3. Lane/Lake
4. Cut/Cup
5. Knit/Sit
6. Pass/Pad
7. Zen/Pen
8. Gain/Game
9. Bank/Sank
10. Set/Get
11. Chair/Fair
12. Hiss/Hit
13. Yacht/Shot
14. Wise/Wine
15. Bin/Fin
16. Feel/Feed
17. Got/Goth
18. Van/Ban
19. Tail/Mail
20. One/Run
21. Nose/Note
22. Let/Less
23. Zone/Bone
24. Bad/Bag
25. Dock/Rock
26. Yank/Thank
27. Deep/Leap
28. Hat/Have
29. Scar/Star
30. Keys/Keep
31. Food/Fool
32. Fin/Fit
33. Right/Light
34. Sane/Pane
35. Job/Knob
36. Have/Half
37. Can/Cat
38. Dare/Chair
39. Dial/While
40. Test/Vest
41. Hope/Pope
42. Sip/Tip
43. Deal/Steal
44. Guess/Mess
45. Jest/Rest
46. Near/Leer
47. Sleet/Sleek
48. Wish/Dish
49. Chip/Chin
50. Camp/Lamp
51. Make/Shake
52. Feet/Seat
53. Hire/Liar
54. Lease/Fleece
55. Press/Dress
56. Tray/Fray
57. Zoom/Doom
58. Hail/Hair
59. Steal/Peal
60. Which/Rich

> **MOTOR SPEECH**

Motor Speech Impairments

Common motor speech impairments include:

APRAXIA OF SPEECH. A speech disorder caused by damage to the part of the brain that coordinates the movements of speech. A person with apraxia has difficulty coordinating what they want to say clearly and consistently.

DYSARTHRIA. A speech disorder caused by weakness of the muscles that help us speak. This weakness comes from an underlying neurological disorder (e.g., stroke, ALS, Parkinson's Disease). Speech may sound unclear, mumbled, or slurred.

MOTOR SPEECH

Intelligibility Tips

Use these tips if people have a hard time understanding what you are saying.

SIGNAL THE START. Let your listener know when you're about to start talking. You can lift your hand, make eye contact, write it down, etc.

NAME THE TOPIC. Say 2-3 words to set your topic.
- *For example, "dinner tonight" or "nephew's birthday."*

KEEP IT SIMPLE. Use easier words and sentence structures.

USE GESTURES. Point, use hand gestures, shrug, shake your head, use facial expressions, etc. to help make your point.

SIGNAL THE END. Avoid interruptions by holding up one finger. Signal when you're finished by holding out your palm to the listener.

USE AN ALPHABET BOARD. An alphabet board is a simple paper with the alphabet written on it. Point to the first letter of every word that you say. Your listener listens to you speak while watching the alphabet board.
- See page 569 for a copy of an alphabet board.

MOTOR SPEECH

Listener Tips

Use these tips if you have a hard time understanding what a loved one is saying.

GIVE YOUR FULL ATTENTION. Listen and watch the entire time the person is speaking.

CONFIRM THE TOPIC. Check that you and the speaker are both on the same topic (ASHA, 2021b).
- "Are we still talking about…?"

USE KEYWORDS. Refer back to words the speaker said to try to create a full narrative.
- "You said dinner. Were you talking about dinner with your family next week?"

ENCOURAGE WRITING, DRAWING, OR GESTURING.

REPEAT EACH WORD. If the speaker is especially hard to understand, repeat each word they say. Confirm that each word is correct before moving on to the next word.

SET GROUND RULES. To avoid frustration, have a set number of times the speaker tries to say something before they take a break or using AAC.

MOTOR SPEECH

Clear Speech Strategies

TALK BIG.
- Over-articulate.

TALK LOUD.
- Increase your volume.

TALK SHORT.
- Take breaths more often; insert pauses every few words.

MOTOR SPEECH

Inspiratory Checking

Use this technique if you "run out of air" while you speak (Netsell, 1998).

INHALE AS DEEPLY AS POSSIBLE. Hold for a few seconds.
- Notice how "big" you feel in your lungs and stomach before breathing out slowly.

INHALE 50% OF YOUR MAXIMUM AMOUNT. Let the air out slowly.

INHALE 50% AGAIN. Inhale to 50% before each sentence, then let the air out slowly while speaking. Fill in the blanks:
- My name is…
- Today's date is…
- The weather today is…
- For breakfast, I ate…
- My favorite holiday is…

CONTINUE PRACTICING. Read menus, newspaper articles, and other reading material aloud. Use this technique when speaking with others.

MOTOR SPEECH

Diaphragmatic Breathing

The diaphragm is a large, dome-shaped muscle under your lungs that plays an important role in breathing. When you breathe in, your diaphragm moves down. This gives your lungs more room to fill with air. Learning to control the movement of your diaphragm can help you produce a louder voice without feeling breathless (Jewell, 2018).

---

1. Put one hand on your stomach and your other hand on your chest. Feel your stomach rise and fall with each breath. Continue for one minute.
   - When you **breathe in**: Your stomach pushes out. The hand on your chest should remain still.
   - When you **breathe out**: Tighten your stomach muscles and feel them pull in. The hand on your chest should remain still.
2. Breathe in, feeling your stomach push out. As you breathe out, say the following sounds and words, remaining aware of your stomach slowly pulling in.
   - Start with simple sounds like "sss" and "shhh."
   - Gradually work up to vowel sounds like "ahh" and "ooh."
   - Work up to say single words like "hello" and your first name.
   - Gradually work up towards longer words, phrases, and sentences.
3. Try to use diaphragmatic breathing throughout the day whenever you speak with someone.

MOTOR SPEECH

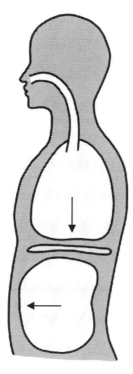 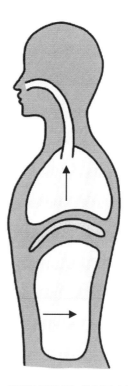

BREATHE IN. Your diaphragm presses down, allowing your lungs to expand. Your stomach pushes out.

BREATHE OUT. Your diaphragm relaxes up and gets smaller. Your stomach goes in.

Breath Control

This exercise helps you take deep enough breaths for speech. It also helps coordinate breathing.

---

1. Breathe in slowly for 3 seconds.
2. Hold your breath for 3 seconds *(Gotter, 2020)*.
3. Release the air slowly for 3 seconds.
4. Continue breathing in this controlled manner.
5. Now, when you exhale, **hold out** these sounds *(Rosenbek & LaPointe, 1985)* for as long as you can:
   - hhh
   - sss
   - thhh
   - fff
   - shhh
6. Now, add vowels to the end of the sounds and **hold them out** for as long as you can:
   - hhha, hhhoe, hhhi, hhhow, whho
   - sssah, ssso, sssee, sssow, sssue
   - thhhaw, thhho, thhhee, thhhow, thhhew
   - fffa, fffoe, fffee, fffow, fffoo
   - shhha, shhhow, shhhe, shhhaow, shhhoe

MOTOR SPEECH

Page 2 of 2

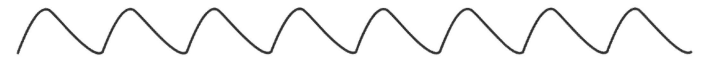

REST BREATHING. Inhale and exhale last about the same amount of time.

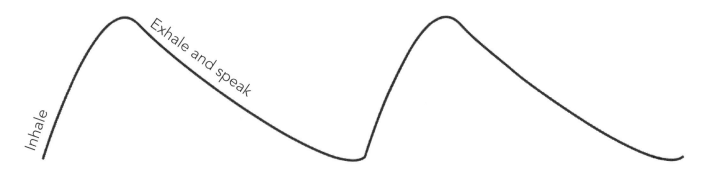

SPEECH BREATHING. Speech breathing is deeper than rest breathing. Exhale is slow and controlled.

MOTOR SPEECH

Building Up Breath Control

Use your breath support strategies while saying the following. You may take breaths as needed.

---

1. Who, what, where, when, why, how.
2. Monday, Tuesday, Wednesday, Thursday, Friday, Saturday, Sunday.
3. One, two, three, four, five, six, seven, eight, nine, ten.
4. Mercury, Venus, Earth, Mars, Jupiter, Saturn, Uranus, Neptune, *Pluto*.
5. January, February, March, April, May, June, July, August, September, October, November, December.
6. His foe thought she was sad.
7. Therapy on Fridays should help.
8. She had three soft feathers.
9. Signs and shapes were found on the foggy hill.
10. Somehow, the frozen shake was half thawed.
11. Jack and Jill went up the hill to fetch a pail of water. Jack fell down and broke his crown and Jill came tumbling after.
12. Mary, Mary, quite contrary, how does your garden grow? With silver bells and cockleshells and pretty maids all in a row.

MOTOR SPEECH

Alphabet Board

A simple alphabet board can greatly improve your intelligibility (how much people can understand your speech). See page 569 for an alphabet board you can copy.

HOW TO USE AN ALPHABET BOARD.
1. Point to the first letter of every word that you say.
2. The listener listens to you speak while watching the alphabet board.

INCREASE INTELLIGIBILITY. When you point to a letter, it gives your listener a written cue. This can help them understand what you're trying to say.

REDUCE SPEECH RATE (A.K.A. PACING BOARD). Pointing to letters helps you to slow down how fast you talk, say each word more clearly, and pause between words *(Van Nuffelen et al., 2009)*.

MOTOR SPEECH

Phone Calls

Say: "To practice your speech strategies, let's pretend to talk on the phone. Pretend that you're calling to…"

Increase the challenge by role-playing. Pretend to answer the phone and ask follow-up questions. For example, "Dr. Merry's office, May speaking… What day of the week works best for you?… I have a 10 am or a 4 pm slot… Has your insurance changed?… Have a great day!"

1. Schedule a dentist appointment for a routine cleaning
2. Order take-out from a Chinese restaurant
3. Ask a sports store about their stock of camping gear
4. Pay a phone bill
5. Confirm your car insurance policy coverage
6. Determine the local library's hours
7. Schedule a salon or barbershop appointment
8. Speak to a technician about a computer issue
9. Order your favorite pizza
10. Book a hotel room for tonight
11. Get directions to a dentist's office
12. Report unfamiliar charges on your credit card bill
13. Tell your doctor that you will be late for your appointment
14. Determine whether a local store is open on the next holiday
15. Ask about an usually large utility bill
16. Confirm the instructions on your prescription bottle
17. Report a power outage in your neighborhood

MOTOR SPEECH

Conversation

Say: "Tell me at least two pros and two cons of…"

1. Living in Hawaii
2. Having ten children
3. Being a vegetarian
4. Wearing school uniforms
5. Using standardized tests in schools
6. Having universal health care
7. Having the ability to fly
8. Advancements in medical technology
9. Shopping online versus in-store
10. Having a local zoo
11. Sending astronauts to Mars
12. Drilling for oil in America
13. Unpaid internships
14. Streaming services, like Netflix and Hulu, versus cable television
15. Free college tuition
16. Social media, like Facebook and Twitter
17. Buying fast food
18. Buying cellphones for children
19. Increasing minimum wage by 50%
20. Making recycling a requirement in all homes

MOTOR SPEECH

Interview

Say: "To practice your speech strategies, let's pretend that you're interviewing for a job. Assume that you have an excellent chance of being hired."

1. Tell me about yourself.
2. What are your strengths?
3. What are your weaknesses?
4. What is something you've put off that you'd like to complete in the coming year?
5. What was your first paid job?
6. What is your dream job?
7. What is your earliest childhood memory?
8. What are your five-year goals? They can be personal or professional.
9. How would you resolve a conflict between you and a coworker?
10. Who are your role models?
11. How would your family and friends describe you?
12. What is your favorite book? Why?
13. What personal or professional achievement are you most proud of?
14. Why should I give you this job?
15. If you could give your 30-year-old self any piece of advice, what would it be?
16. What advice would you give to your most recent boss?
17. How do you handle criticism?
18. What 5 items would you bring to a deserted island?

MOTOR SPEECH

Monologues

Say: "I'm going to give you a topic to talk about for 3-5 minutes. You will have about a minute to prepare."

1. A previous career
2. How to get started with a hobby
3. A book plot summary
4. Your childhood
5. Your family
6. The most memorable TV commercial you've seen
7. The most beautiful place you've ever been
8. Your most recent dream
9. The most delicious meal you've ever had
10. How to learn to cook
11. Your dream house
12. Your best friend
13. How to plan a road trip
14. What to do during a natural disaster
15. How to throw a dinner party
16. How to make new friends
17. How to sleep better at night
18. How to make a homemade gift (e.g. baked goods)
19. The perfect weekend
20. Your role model

Sentence Stress

*Prosody, the melody line of speech, is important for clear communication. To improve your prosody, emphasize the bold word in each sentence. Emphasize the word by speaking it **louder** and with a **higher pitch** than the other words. **Exaggerate** as much as you can! Try using a sing-song voice, like a school teacher.*

---

1. How are **YOU**?
   How **ARE** you?
   HOW are you?

2. Where **IS** she?
   Where is **SHE**?
   WHERE is she?

3. I don't **KNOW**.
   I don't know.
   I **DON'T** know.

4. What a **FUNNY** story!
   WHAT a funny story!
   What a funny **STORY**!

5. **WHAT** a lovely day.
   What a **LOVELY** day.
   What a lovely **DAY**.

MOTOR SPEECH

6. I **CAN'T** believe it!
   I can't believe it!
   I can't **BELIEVE** it!

7. It's the third house on the **RIGHT**.
   It's the **THIRD** house on the right.
   It's the third **HOUSE** on the right.

8. He **BOUGHT** a new car.
   He bought a **NEW** car.
   He bought a new **CAR**.

9. **PLEASE** turn off the lights.
   Please turn off the **LIGHTS**.
   Please turn **OFF** the lights.

10. It was a traditional **WEDDING**.
    It **WAS** a traditional wedding.
    It was a **TRADITIONAL** wedding.

11. I hope I **GET** the job.
    I hope I get the **JOB**.
    I **HOPE** I get the job.

12. My **FLIGHT** is tomorrow morning.
    My flight is **TOMORROW** morning.
    MY flight is tomorrow morning.

MOTOR SPEECH

13. Does **ANYONE** know where it is?
    DOES anyone know where it is?
    Does anyone know **WHERE** it is?

14. She's even older than **ME**!
    SHE'S even older than me!
    She's even **OLDER** than me!

15. Wash your **HANDS** with soap and warm water.
    Wash your hands with **SOAP** and warm water.
    Wash your hands with soap and **WARM** water.

16. I **NEED** to arrive at the hospital by 5 am.
    I need to arrive at the hospital by **5 AM**.
    I need to **ARRIVE** at the hospital by 5 am.

17. **YOU'RE** the best speech therapist ever!
    You're the **BEST** speech therapist ever!
    You're the best speech therapist **EVER**!

18. Turn **LEFT** at the light.
    TURN left at the light.
    Turn left at the **LIGHT**.

MOTOR SPEECH

Heteronyms

*Prosody, the melody line of speech, is important for clear communication. Heteronyms are words that are spelled the same but are stressed or pronounced differently. Improve your prosody by emphasizing the bold heteronym in each sentence. Emphasize by increasing the **loudness** and **pitch** of your voice. **Exaggerate** as much as possible!*

---

1. The **subject** was pretty boring.
   Please don't **subject** me to math.

2. Let's **resume** the interview.
   I need to submit my **resume** for the job.

3. Please **relay** my message to your boss.
   The project was a **relay** race of tasks.

4. She can be such a **rebel** when she's angry.
   She will **rebel** when she hears the bad news.

5. I held the **record** for the race for five years.
   Please **record** my time in the official books.

6. The store's **produce** is so fresh.
   The manager can **produce** such great results.

MOTOR SPEECH

7. The **present** was thoughtful and sweet.
   She will **present** it beautifully.

8. Can you really **permit** such an act?
   You can buy a **permit** at the front office.

9. The books were in **perfect** alignment.
   She could **perfect** her art if she practiced.

10. I would **object** if it would make a difference.
    I don't want to be the **object** of contempt.

11. He was an **invalid** for many years.
    That contract was **invalid** as of last year.

12. The **incense** gave off a subtle, pleasant smell.
    Don't **incense** her by insulting her dog.

13. The meal was easy to **digest** after drinking a cup of water.
    The local printed **digest** was easy to read.

14. I'll **desert** you here if you touch my radio again.
    The gas mileage in the **desert** is always a little worse.

15. They'll **convict** you straightaway if you don't prepare your defense.
    They say that the **convict** had escaped for 3 hours.

16. I am definitely a **convert** to your coffee shop.
    Please don't try to **convert** me to tea.

17. I'm not willing to sign your **contract** if you don't allow me to read it.
    I can't be sure I won't **contract** the flu.

18. He was **content** with a comfy armchair and a full pantry.
    His life held little **content** besides waking up, eating, and sleeping.

19. The police will **conduct** an investigation soon.
    The way attitude influences our **conduct** is very clear.

20. We can **attribute** our success to her commitment.
    Her **attribute** of gumption made the program successful.

22. The large **console** was meant to look flashy.
    I had to **console** my friend when her car broke down.

23. It will take at least a week to **deliberate** on the decision.
    I scheduled the massage in a **deliberate** attempt to relax.

24. He hopes to **lead** his troops to victory.
    The troops dodged the **lead** cannonballs.

25. Is there an **alternate** route to the beach?
    I **alternate** between staying in traffic and returning home.

MOTOR SPEECH

Phonemic Lists

For patients with acquired apraxia of speech. Use the Phonemic Lists to target specific phonemes by position and length.

The lists are organized in the following order:
- Initial position monosyllabic, bisyllabic, and multisyllabic words
- Medial and final position words
- Initial, medial, and final position sentences

MOTOR SPEECH

/p/ initial

Paw	Peek	Parking	Pelican
Pay	Pace	Painful	Porcelain
Pee	Peel	Polite	Piano
Poo	Pink	Peaceful	Pioneer
Pot	Pour	Package	Policy
Pole	Pave	Pushy	Pollution
Page	Pox	Pooling	Podium
Peace	Pause	Piled	Poetry
Peer	Polly	Painter	Position
Puck	Pierce	Palace	Projection
Pig	Potter	Punish	Prejudice
Pet	Police	Pursue	Primary
Pass	Polar	Pretend	Prodigy
Park	Panic	Prison	Processor
Pen	Puzzle	Pony	Provider
Pull	Poodle	Privately	Pulverize
Pain	Paddle	Piracy	Pyramid
Pooch	Pencil	Perfectly	Panicky
Ping	Pocket	Promising	Purify
Pack	Patient	Politics	Potato
Pod	Pollute	Panama	
Poof	Parent	Pentagon	

/p/ medial & final

Apple	Saucepan	Hardship
Slippers	Lipstick	Backslap
Hippo	Supper	Blacktop
Grumpy	Grapefruit	Bullwhip
Teapot	Jumping	Asleep
Diaper	Copy	Bishop
Shampoo	Tipsy	Barhop
Open	Sleeping	Lineup
Zipper	Helpful	Mockup
Happy	Hippie	Mishap
Dropper	Internship	Hiccup
Mopping	Barbershop	Gossip
Important	Develop	Turnip
Airport	Shortstop	Teacup
Camping	Eavesdrop	Workup
Apart	Fingertip	Yelp
Staple	Photoshop	Tarp
Shapes	Follow-up	Soap
Apron	Handicap	Ramp
Notepad	Backflip	

MOTOR SPEECH

/p/ sentences

1. The pushy politician put the pencil on the paper.
2. Please prepare the pudding from the package.
3. Place the Peace Prize on the podium.
4. Pretend the prancing pony is pink.
5. Pass the pepper to my plate.
6. The potatoes and pumpkin pie are picturesque.
7. Pace your pedaling to preserve your power.
8. That person is a painter and poet.
9. My peaceful parents like to party pretty hard.
10. Plenty of puppies play pretend.

MOTOR SPEECH

/b/ initial

Bay	Bass	Bachelor	Basically
Boo	Bite	Backlight	Biology
Boy	Best	Baffle	Backhanded
Bye	Boss	Basic	Behavior
Be	Bar	Bedroom	Benefit
Bow	Bank	Beggar	Boundary
Back	Bought	Bloody	Boloney
Bake	Baker	Boil	Bravado
Beak	Buffer	Bottom	Bookseller
Bed	Buoyant	Breakfast	Beginner
Bash	Bitter	Bucket	Battleship
Beef	Blizzard	British	Battery
Big	Boutique	Barren	Busier
Bag	Below	Blister	Buttermilk
Bog	Berry	Bandage	Bulldozer
Ball	Better	Bicycle	Brilliant
Bam	Birthday	Butterfly	Bronchitis
Beam	Bottle	Banana	Boulevard
Bin	Baggage	Buffalo	Bashfully
Best	Breathy	Bifocal	
Bore	Boyish	Bravo	
Beer	Balloon	Beautiful	

MOTOR SPEECH

/b/ medial & final

Above	Zebra	Club
Raspberry	Cowboy	Knob
Embezzle	Cutback	Curb
Jukebox	Anybody	Verb
Kickboxer	Crumbly	Crab
Object	Chamber	Glib
Zombie	Capable	Swab
Checkbook	Cymbals	Grab
Matchbox	Eyeball	Herb
Fabric	Affable	Snub
Herbal	Corncob	Dab
Emblazon	Adverb	Slob
Textbook	Superb	Stub
Chubby	Absorb	Drab
Lockbox	Squib	Jab
Gazebo	Celeb	Dub
Subject	Scrub	Fib
Abject	Rehab	Blab
Flyby	Throb	Nub
Jumbo	Cob	Fab

/b/ sentences

MOTOR SPEECH

1. By breakfast, the baby was bawling.
2. Because of the break, the boys went bowling.
3. Brighten the bedroom by building a balcony.
4. The best bookseller for board books is in Boston.
5. Beating the best in the business was a burden.
6. The buttermilk biscuits at brunch were a blast.
7. Before we begin, let's break bread with the boss.
8. Believe me, the biologist bought the bacteria.
9. Get the best base price by bartering from the beginning.
10. The bachelor brings bravado and brevity to the buffet.

MOTOR SPEECH

/m/ initial

Me	Make	Mitten	Manual
My	Month	Moral	Marrying
Mow	Man	Mini	Medicate
May	Must	Minor	Mineral
Ma	Main	Major	Miracle
Moo	Mouth	Marvel	Misery
Meat	Moon	Master	Microphone
Maze	Might	Molar	Mislabel
Move	Mayor	Mercy	Mitigate
More	Motor	Muffin	Microwave
Met	Monday	Mobile	Modify
Mean	Mother	Mountaineer	Molecule
Mall	Mirror	Monster	Mosquito
Mage	Movie	Mister	Mobilize
Mile	Mullet	Mustard	Motivate
Mate	Mower	Minimal	Mutual
Mint	Music	Multitude	Mutiny
Mole	Muzzle	Melody	Mystery
Milk	Modest	Meteor	Mythical
Most	Meager	Mechanic	Motherly
Mix	Mission	Majesty	
Mad	Mighty	Manicure	

MOTOR SPEECH

/m/ medial & final

Homey	Formal	Storm
Communicate	Flamboyant	Feminism
Jackhammer	Amphibian	Platform
Amber	Benchmark	Bathroom
Checkmark	Cinemas	Mushroom
Example	Harmony	Warm
Number	Amazing	Kilogram
Bemuse	Jumpy	Sarcasm
Sympathy	Humpty	Exclaim
Champion	Alarm	System
Symmetry	Bloom	Bottom
Empathy	Broom	Podium
Framing	Charm	Anthem
Lumberjack	Cream	Disarm
Squeamish	Flame	Prism
Vampire	Realm	
Homogenized	Auditorium	
Victimize	Criticism	
Women	Classroom	
Computer	Petroleum	
Decimal	Film	

MOTOR SPEECH

/m/ sentences

1. Maybe the monk makes moscato.
2. Must we move to Montana on Monday?
3. My manager makes magnificent muffins.
4. My mom married mean Mr. Mustard.
5. The muzzle made the mutt mutter more.
6. My major is math, and it makes me mad.
7. The mountaineer marked the mount with a mighty mound.
8. Each mythical monster moves marvelously.
9. The microscope's messages were mislabeled.
10. We visit Maryland in May for mini vacations.

MOTOR SPEECH

/w/ initial

Whoa	Wort	Willow	Whispering
We	Wife	Wildlife	Wisconsin
Why	Walk	Wasted	Wolverine
Whim	Whiz	Winner	Wonderland
Wish	Web	Wizard	Wellbeing
Wig	Witch	Walrus	Withstanding
Wide	Weed	Whisky	Wistfully
Wad	Wonder	Whistle	Walloping
Wade	Water	Worthy	Worsening
Woof	Woman	Wardrobe	Worthiness
Wag	Winter	Whiskers	Watering
Whack	Welcome	Weasel	Wackily
Wall	Wisdom	Weapon	Wanderlust
Womb	Wishful	Whiten	Wheelbarrow
One	Whisper	Wanted	Worshipping
Win	Waffle	Washington	Wireless
Whip	Worry	Weathering	Wildflower
Wipe	Without	Wonderful	Whatever
Wore	Working	Withering	Wimbledon
Wax	Weekend	Warrior	Wallflower
Ways	Weary	Weightlifting	
Worm	Western	Waterfall	

MOTOR SPEECH

/w/ medial

- Dour
- Sour
- Power
- Shower
- Tower
- Flower
- Homework
- Towel
- Awake
- Lower
- Sewing
- Owl
- Sandwich
- Showing
- Awkward

- Always
- Highway
- Someone
- Reward
- Nationwide
- Nowadays
- Microwave
- Sidewalk
- Awarded
- Awakened
- Hour
- Sunflower
- Devour
- Foul

/w/ sentences

1. Why wonder what will happen?
2. Well-wishers won't weaken the worst of my worries.
3. When I want a waffle, I walk to Wanda's.
4. We will win weightlifting this weekend.
5. The wife filled the wheelbarrow with wild weeds.
6. He white-washed the withering walls for the walk-through.
7. The western wardrobe is worn with one Winchester.
8. Washington winters are wet and windy.
9. I went to the wharf for the whisky and water.
10. Without the water, we'll waver and wither.

MOTOR SPEECH

/f/ initial

Fee	Fib	Forget	Firework
Foe	Fad	Fallen	Festival
Fill	Fork	Feather	Fireman
Fan	Far	Female	Furious
Fog	False	Fury	Fundraiser
Food	Four	Foolish	Federal
Fish	Flop	Flatten	Flexible
Fizz	Flea	Fairy	Forbidden
Fix	Feeling	Farmer	Flammable
Fin	Fourteen	Finance	Fortunate
Fat	Friday	Flavor	Finalist
Fought	Father	Flashlight	Faculty
Feed	Football	Freeway	Fingerprint
Feel	Forest	Futon	Fictional
Free	Famous	Fitness	Forgiving
Fresh	Fashion	Family	Firewall
Flip	Flower	Favorite	Following
Fox	Finger	Feminine	Feminist
Frog	Fountain	Forever	Forgotten
Fear	Final	Factory	Forgery
Phone	Frozen	Fantasy	Funnily
Fawn	Focus	Formula	

MOTOR SPEECH

/f/ medial & final

Coffee	Quantify	Rough
Professor	Defrost	Skiff
Effect	Sulfur	Decaf
Superficial	After	Pilaf
Official	Crawfish	Stuff
Reflexive	Difficult	Off
Justify	Prefix	Handcuff
Qualify	Muffin	Triumph
Liquefy	Earmuff	Calf
Inflexible	Showoff	Carafe
Affable	Bailiff	Laugh
Chieftain	Wolf	Staff
Chiffon	Sheriff	Behalf
Efficacy	Cuff	Choreograph
Heffalump	Belief	Giraffe
Befuddle	Itself	Telegraph
Traffic	Relief	
Joyful	Roof	
Backflow	Housewife	
Chaffing	Cliff	

MOTOR SPEECH

/f/ sentences

1. First find the photo of the fresh flowers.
2. The fingerprint was found by the front foyer.
3. The forest feels like freedom to my fettered mind.
4. I'd forgotten the fee for the founding fundraiser.
5. There's frozen fish and other food in the freezer.
6. Filming begins on the first Friday of February.
7. The factory was financed by funds from the fashionista.
8. The footballer felt his fibula fracture.
9. The full-grown flamingos in Florida took flight.
10. Facing the fact that the photo was a forgery made me feel forlorn.

MOTOR SPEECH

/v/ initial

Vow	Volley	Verbose	Virtual
Vote	Value	Voter	Visible
Voice	Villain	Verbal	Visiting
Van	Vision	Vanquish	Viaduct
Vet	Vacuum	Venting	Vanishing
Vat	Vintage	Vocal	Vagabond
Veer	Vessel	Vainly	Vertebrae
Vine	Veto	Viewer	Veracity
View	Vapor	Violence	Visceral
Vice	Venture	Vanilla	Vertical
Vox	Viper	Volleyball	Visitor
Verb	Venue	Volcano	Verify
Void	Vineyard	Victory	Various
Veal	Venom	Vacation	Vertigo
Vogue	Visit	Viola	Vegetable
Vamp	Valid	Veteran	Vendetta
Vague	Vibrate	Vitamin	Validate
Volt	Valet	Vanity	
Vest	Vanish	Vehicle	
Vase	Visor	Vinegar	

MOTOR SPEECH

/v/ medial & final

Overt
Equivalent
Civil
Overpriced
Civilized
Rival
Shaving
Approval
Every
Fever
Device
Everywhere
Feverish
Loving
Behavior
Extrovert
Heaven
Seven
Juvenile

Jovial
Impoverish
Observation
Rejuvenate
Shoveling
Wavelength
Avalanche
Privacy
Improv
Love
Cave
Dove
Wave
Five
Halve
Serve
Live
Glove
Weave

Trove
Naive
Grove
Octave
Remove
Relive
Starve
Active
Native
Absolve
Explosive
Missive
Achieve
Deceive
Elective
Adhesive
Cohesive
Beehive

MOTOR SPEECH

/v/ sentences

1. Veterans in Virginia vote for their values.
2. The vineyard vetted very valuable vintage Vermouth.
3. The vaccines for the virus varied in validity.
4. The vibrato of her voice was vague and vapid.
5. The Vikings vanquished the vagabonds during the volley.
6. I take various vitamins and eat vegetables to validate my vanity.
7. Her venom vindicated my valiant vendetta.
8. The vat of vinegar vanished on Valentine's Day.
9. I visited, drove a vehicle to the volcano, and viewed from the vantage point.
10. The violets and verbena were vibrant in the vase.

MOTOR SPEECH

"th" initial

The	Thaw	Thicken	Thermostat
This	Thing	Thrilling	Thunderstruck
That	Thick	Threefold	Thoughtfully
Though	Thumb	Thermal	Thickening
Then	Third	Thriving	Thoroughfare
They	Thank	Threadbare	Thrombosis
There	Thud	Thickness	Throwaway
Them	Thirst	Thumbprint	Thoroughly
These	Therefore	Thorny	Theorize
Than	Themselves	Throwback	Thinkable
Thought	Therein	Throbbing	Thermally
Through	Thorough	Thumbtack	Theatric
Three	Throughout	Thicket	Thunderstorm
Thrash	Thirty	Thumbing	Thriftiness
Threat	Thirsty	Thieving	Thespian
Thrill	Thoughtful	Thinner	Thenceforward
Thread	Thursday	Therewithal	Three-quarters
Thief	Thunder	Therewithin	Thievishness
Thug	Thousand	Theater	Thoughtfulness
Throw	Thirteen	Therapy	Thinkingly
Thorn	Thrifty	Thanksgiving	Theorizing
Thin	Thimble	Thankfulness	

MOTOR SPEECH

"th" medial & final

Birthing	Nothing	Truth
Bother	Panther	Beneath
Dither	Rethread	Stealth
Father	Seething	Mammoth
Mother	Pathetic	With
Leather	Smoothie	Faith
Weather	Sympathy	Health
Worthy	Withdrew	Growth
Athletes	Withdraw	Wealth
Amethyst	Youthful	Smooth
Author	Fifth	Breath
Bathrobe	Birth	Hearth
Bathtub	Length	Sleuth
Earthy	Smith	Zenith
Ethereal	Cloth	North
Ethics	Math	South
Faithful	Labyrinth	Tenth
Loathsome	Mouth	Width
Method	Both	
Motherly	Strength	

MOTOR SPEECH

"th" sentences

1. The thief thwarted the sleuth.
2. The smoothie in the thermos was thirst-quenching.
3. They gathered thirty threadbare thespians in the theatre.
4. Thanksgiving is now the third Thursday of the month.
5. I'm thinner although my width is thickening.
6. The thick thicket was thoroughly thriving with thorns.
7. The weather to the north calls for three thunderstorms.
8. The therapist thinks it's a worthy method.
9. This and that are more than nothing.
10. I theorize that you'll thank me for thinking ahead.

MOTOR SPEECH

/d/ initial

Do	Dare	Dual	Defender
Doe	Door	Dashboard	Disagree
Da	Date	Disguise	Dominance
Die	Dawn	Dairy	Dubious
Day	Diet	Delay	Domino
Doll	Dolphin	Dwelling	Dialogue
Dug	Dancing	Debut	Decibel
Doze	Donkey	Depot	Disengage
Deck	Daisy	Dangerous	Desire
Ditch	Daily	Depression	Disarming
Dine	Daughter	Dinosaur	Durable
Dab	Dinner	Discipline	Dispenser
Dog	Double	Delicious	
Dock	Doing	Discover	
Dance	Design	Dignity	
Dope	Demo	Diary	
Dome	Dollar	Difference	
Dill	Despair	Delicate	
Dip	Discuss	Division	
Dire	Delight	Diploma	
Does	Denim	Discussion	
Dice	Diesel	Deliver	

MOTOR SPEECH

/d/ medial & final

Leader
Jeopardy
Paddy
Rider
Merchandise
Hazardous
Prejudice
Oxidize
Bedroom
Shadow
Humidity
Backdoor
Midsize
Stardom
Kingdom
Zodiac
Haddock
Border
Skydive

Exceeds
Heyday
Holiday
Ladybug
Midweek
Padlock
Paradox
Food
Bread
Bird
Head
Salad
Friend
Road
Blizzard
Broad
Centipede
Lampshade
Platitude

Downside
Slide
Attitude
Persuade
Coincide
Homemade
Renegade
Degrade
Provide
Commode
Implode
Second
Allude
Chide
Secede
Parade
Florid

MOTOR SPEECH

/d/ sentences

1. Don't you dare delay this discussion.
2. The deacon died with dignity.
3. Dancing with dinosaurs is a dangerous endeavor.
4. Deliver the disclaimer without delay.
5. The double date was dour and depressing.
6. Dodging dialogue is desired for diplomacy.
7. Dad was disagreeable about driving in the dark.
8. Do the dogs dare guard the road?
9. The damaging discourse was disastrous to the defendant.
10. Dice and dominos were displayed in the doorway.

MOTOR SPEECH

/t/ initial

Two	Tear	Teamwork	Typical
Toe	Twig	Tummy	Terrible
Tie	Term	Talking	Temperature
Top	Toll	Topper	Tambourine
Type	Twirl	Taxi	Tidily
Toy	Tick	Towel	Tapestry
Touch	Taco	Tempo	Turbulent
Tap	Talent	Teller	Takeaway
Tee	Turkey	Tofu	Ticklish
Tip	Toilet	Temple	Taskmaster
Tool	Teacher	Typo	Tipsiness
Time	Table	Tether	Tampering
Tin	Twelve	Taker	Taxable
Tuck	Tulip	Teenager	Tedious
Tone	Tuesday	Together	Takeover
Teach	Tattle	Tomorrow	Topical
Tooth	Tuba	Tobacco	Terrific
Tire	Tiger	Telescope	
Task	Twinkle	Tourism	
Tell	Toothbrush	Twiddling	
Twill	Tucker	Temperate	
Ton	Temper	Tibia	

MOTOR SPEECH

/t/ medial & final

Empty	Atone	Print
Utensil	Abducted	Floret
Valentine	Detox	Skillet
Military	Antiques	Artifact
Hunter	Canister	Corset
Guitar	Feast	Destruct
Bathtub	East	Flirt
Hotel	West	Forecast
Jointly	Wet	Bat
Montana	Debt	Insolent
Futon	Guilt	Cast
Fistful	Strict	Viaduct
Depicted	Bigfoot	Covenant
Hotly	Blunt	Deposit
Unity	Chauvinist	Supplement
Retired	Circuit	Convenient
Sting	Chemist	
Stupid	Collect	

MOTOR SPEECH

/t/ sentences

1. Toddlers tend to tax my tolerance.
2. My tuba teacher was a taskmaster.
3. I took the taxi to town on Tuesday.
4. The bathtub was empty each time.
5. The tap is in the toolbox next to the outlet.
6. I took two minutes off my time and tied!
7. The twins teamed up to take the lead.
8. Typing with your toes is tormenting.
9. The tune was all toots and tones.
10. She tiptoes like a tiger in tulips.

MOTOR SPEECH

/n/ initial

No	Nurse	Nickel	Nevermore
New	Numb	Nephew	Nauseous
Now	Nail	Normal	Neighborhood
Gnaw	Niece	Nosey	Newcomer
Knee	Nape	Nibble	Noisily
Nope	Knoll	Necklace	Nasally
Nil	Nymph	Nasal	Nursery
Nay	Norse	Notion	Narrowly
Nap	Knot	Neither	Numeral
Nick	Neo	Noble	Neurosis
Nab	Naive	Neglect	Numbering
Knack	Naked	Nausea	Neighborly
Knock	Nature	Nimble	Newspaper
Kneel	Nothing	Navel	Namesake
Name	Number	Namely	Narrowing
Gnome	Never	Novel	Newsworthy
Nor	Nuclear	Nipple	Neutralize
Nare	Nova	Natural	Narcissism
Near	Narrow	November	Nervously
Nose	Nightmare	Nemesis	
North	Navy	Nobody	
Noise	Nemo	Nebula	

MOTOR SPEECH

/n/ medial & final

Sunny	Cognitive	Again
Dinner	Quenched	Rotten
Honey	Kindly	Violin
Vanilla	Cunning	Falcon
Piano	Conquer	Carbon
Tennis	Juniper	Thrown
Funny	Peanut	Sudden
Animal	Quantity	Screen
Confuse	Mining	Broken
Tent	Journey	Remain
Banjo	Rain	Design
Ensure	Amen	Balloon
Injury	Darn	Tuition
Frenzy	Oxen	Cushion
Spinning	Oxygen	Fifteen
Tenure	Sedan	Meridian
Twenty	Raven	Stubborn
Many	Queen	Corn
Pancake	Plain	Phone
Analyze	Brown	

MOTOR SPEECH

/n/ sentences

1. I nearly nabbed the new newspaper.
2. The knight kneeled before his nemesis.
3. The necklace needs new nickel ornaments.
4. Needless to say, he never knew my name.
5. The nightmare of a nuclear attack made me nervous.
6. It's natural for a newborn to be noisy.
7. She had a knack for knotting the net.
8. The neighbor's nosiness was noteworthy.
9. My knee has never been so numb.
10. The nimble niece knew her numbers.

MOTOR SPEECH

/s/ initial

See	Sell	Second	Several
So	Sale	Service	Sangria
Sue	Some	Subject	Sunflower
Saw	Sun	Struggle	Sleepover
Say	Sore	Soda	Signature
Sick	Sat	Standard	Silicon
Stick	Save	Sweater	Superman
Stock	Says	Stable	Sacrifice
Slay	Snicker	Skinny	Studio
Slim	Soldier	Saga	Snorkeling
Sip	Safety	Style	Surrender
Stove	Slightly	Siren	Samurai
Sap	Stutter	Syndrome	Survival
Sob	Steeply	Seashell	Symmetry
Sack	Snoring	Snowy	Succulent
Sad	Starry	Specter	Strategy
Said	Seven	Sierra	Suddenly
Surf	Secret	Seventy	Selection
Safe	Solid	Syllable	Submarine
Sage	Snowman	Solution	Sombrero
Sag	Sparkle	September	Subjection
Sock	Savage	Stadium	Scholarship

MOTOR SPEECH

/s/ medial & final

Passive
Mistake
Casket
Poster
Blissful
Downsized
Basket
Jigsaw
Mosquito
Mustard
Asset
Excited
Insight
Gaslight
Capsize
Justify
Whisky
Boston
Dissect
Decent
Messy

Joyously
Midsized
Misguided
Basic
Rustle
Consume
Fasting
Intense
Expense
Dress
Horse
Grass
Goose
Kiss
Goddess
Minus
Metrics
Jobless
Hideous
Class
Joyous

Chorus
Radius
Cross
Pelvis
Cactus
Chaos
Abyss
This
Bogus
Tennis
Porous
Painless
Calculus
Robotics
Gracious

MOTOR SPEECH

/s/ sentences

1. Save the sledding and snowmen for snowy days.
2. Stay home from school when you're sick.
3. Sleeping soundly is easier said than done.
4. I slipped the sweater on when the sun set.
5. Several sangrias later, I was snoring sonorously.
6. The syndrome's survival rates skyrocket with the synthetic serum.
7. Several soldiers sat in the stern of the submarine.
8. She said she was selected for the scholarship on Sunday.
9. I would style the skirt with a scarf and simple sunglasses.
10. My strategy to stay skinny is to skip soda and steak.

MOTOR SPEECH

/z/ initial

Zoo	Zipper	Zealand
Zee	Zombie	Zucchini
Zone	Zany	Zillion
Zip	Zeta	Zinnia
Zap	Zeppelin	Zombify
Zig	Ziplock	Zodiac
Zag	Zappy	Zeroing
Zinc	Zipping	Zaniest
Zeal	Zagging	Zaniness
Zoom	Zephyr	Zestfulness
Zilch	Zapper	Zealotry
Zen	Zooming	Zambia
Zing	Zesting	Zesty
Zonk	Zipless	Zeitgeist
Zed	Zenith	Zealander
Zest	Zinger	Xylophone
Zero	Zealous	
Zebra	Zealot	
Zippy	Zonked	
Zelda	Zion	

MOTOR SPEECH

/z/ medial & final

Easy	Sizing	Shoes
Music	Dazzles	Batteries
Puzzle	Dozen	Creatives
Lizard	Hazard	Depresses
Desert	Horizon	Hardwires
Scissors	Nose	Showbiz
Daisy	Stylize	Buzz
Wizard	Prize	Tease
Dessert	Breeze	Phrase
Lazy	Keys	Polarize
Fuzzy	Bees	Supervise
Present	Cheese	Surprise
Razor	Sneeze	Paralyze
Magazine	Shells	Analyze
President	Apologize	Choose
Closet	Toes	Oppose
Gazing	Jazz	Amuse
Bizarre	Gauze	
Buzzing	Gaze	

MOTOR SPEECH

/z/ sentences

1. There are dozens of zombies zooming by.
2. The zealot said zany and bizarre phrases.
3. I apologize that I zonked out during your presentation.
4. The prize-winning pretzel created a lot of buzz.
5. The shoes in the magazine are a zillion dollars.
6. The jazz musician had a dazzling presence.
7. Zion allows zero cars to zip through.
8. The zucchinis are next to the daisies and zinnias.
9. Zest the oranges with a razor or scissors.
10. The showbiz president zoomed in on New Zealand.

MOTOR SPEECH

/ɹ/ initial

Row	Roast	Ruby	Relative
Raw	Rest	Robot	Ratio
Rain	Rev	Reptile	Radiant
Ray	Ram	Recess	Reflection
Reek	Right	Racy	Retina
Rad	Rum	Ribbon	Remedy
Rack	Reach	Realize	Recession
Rod	Rent	Raffle	Revival
Rich	Relish	Respite	Rosary
Rash	Railing	Retail	Reasoning
Raid	Regal	Rapid	Rectangle
Reef	Resting	Rhyming	Replica
Rig	Riddle	Rumble	Radius
Rag	Respect	Repent	Renegade
Rail	Random	Runway	Rapidly
Roll	Riot	Resume	Runaway
Roam	Research	Reaction	Ritual
Rim	Relief	Rodeo	Reliant
Rang	Reject	Royalty	Reflexive
Rap	Raining	Radio	Romantic
Rope	Really	Republic	Respectful
Ripe	Resource	Religion	Radiance

MOTOR SPEECH

/ɹ/ medial & final

Hairy	Workshop	Senior
Phrase	Airborne	Lawyer
Blizzard	Armor	Juniper
Quart	Curable	Power
Exercise	Deodorant	Concur
Hybrid	Orthodox	Liquor
Blueberry	Formula	Amateur
Grizzly	Bearing	Atmosphere
Jargon	Chores	Explore
Ornament	Feverish	Hotwire
Baritone	Fear	Capture
Church	Flour	Empire
Earth	Your	Square
Fortune	Hair	Figure
Hero	Door	Fracture
Memory	Fewer	Mediocre
Flickering	Offer	Conspire
Hardly	Laser	Shore
Spread	Zapper	Nor
Throat	Humor	

MOTOR SPEECH

/ɹ/ sentences

1. I really regret writing the review.
2. The rapid recession made residents reel.
3. I read her resume on reflex.
4. Their richest resource was the ruby.
5. The renegade rapidly ran away.
6. We'll revisit the race in the recording.
7. I'll rest once I'm rich and respected.
8. The religious ritual included robes and a rosary.
9. The reptile rested on a rock in its residence.
10. I'll roam the road in my rugged car.

MOTOR SPEECH

/l/ initial

Lou	Loop	Learning	Lottery
Law	Lag	Lightning	Lemonade
Life	Lace	Lyrics	Limited
Love	Leg	Liter	Lavender
Laugh	Like	Logic	Licensure
Live	Lime	Locker	Licorice
Less	Limb	Looking	Luxury
Long	Loot	Loser	Ligament
Line	Lion	Logger	Liable
Low	Laughter	Leather	Ladybug
Lie	Liar	Larger	Logistics
Lab	Language	Listen	Lunatic
Look	Lady	Lavish	Ludicrous
Lock	Lemon	Limit	Listener
Lee	Loving	Lunar	Lasagna
Lift	Llama	Linear	Lingering
Left	Lava	Legacy	Lenient
Lay	Lobster	Library	Laziness
Light	Later	Liberty	Likable
Lead	Lotion	Lucrative	Lacerate
Leash	Liquid	Lyrical	Laminate
Lip	Lesson	Listening	

MOTOR SPEECH

/l/ medial & final

Yellow	Jobless	Squeal
Silver	Plates	Pummel
Column	Unlucky	Symbol
Puzzling	Zealous	Vowel
Black	Backlot	Nickel
Palace	Buffalo	Shovel
Geology	Helping	Towel
Cycling	Jelly	Betrayal
Complex	Milk	Propel
Slow	Relax	Pencil
Stolen	Graceful	Casual
Exclaim	Blackmail	Hassle
Mailbox	Functional	Fossil
Alchemy	Well	Reveal
Calcium	Haul	Vessel
Resolve	Proximal	Actual
Holiday	Bowl	Recycle
Jawline	Physical	Bubble
Juggled	Decimal	Roll
Mallet	Jail	Mile

MOTOR SPEECH

/l/ sentences

1. You'll likely live a long life.
2. The lasagna came with lettuce and lemonade.
3. It's just my luck that I lost the lottery.
4. The lamp in the living room is leaning to the left.
5. Lift the lever to release the load.
6. Lower the luggage in the locker.
7. The lavender lotion had a lingering smell.
8. Leaving Legos on the lawn is lazy.
9. The leaping lava leveled the lagoon.
10. She lead the lawyers through a lengthy lecture.

MOTOR SPEECH

/k/ initial

Caw	Come	Kidding	Kimono
Cow	King	Careful	Customer
Key	Kiss	Kitchen	Cantaloupe
Cope	Can	Kingdom	Koala
Kid	Catch	Keyboard	Kilowatt
Kite	Coin	Ketchup	Kinetic
Kind	Cone	Kilo	Consonant
Kill	Cold	Kidney	Company
Keep	Candy	Keyhole	Casino
Keen	Candle	Kernel	Curious
Kip	Camel	Keeper	Companion
Kiln	Carrot	Kipper	Confusion
Kept	Cabbage	Kindness	Calcium
Keel	Cabin	Calendar	Carefully
Kilt	Cartoon	Camera	Clarity
Kraft	Color	Capital	Conscience
Corn	Costume	Cardinal	Caramel
Cage	Country	Carpenter	Conference
Cup	Cousin	Colorful	Capable
Cat	Kitten	Computer	Compliment
Count	Catcher	Consider	Copious
Cut	Couple	Correction	

MOTOR SPEECH

/k/ medial & final

Ticket	Checkup	Make
Turkey	Junkmail	Poke
Bacon	Biker	Pancake
Jacket	Backfire	Shake
Bucket	Folksy	Organic
Necklace	Pickup	Chipmunk
Soccer	Wicked	Manic
Breakfast	Bakery	Gigantic
Chicken	Fork	Pitchfork
Looking	Chapstick	Shark
Uncle	Walk	Music
Pocket	Mark	Squeak
Doctor	Embark	Medic
Blackberry	Panic	Black
Circle	Whisk	Knock
Smoky	Chalk	Desk
Jackpot	Shock	Amuck
Joker	Hallmark	Poetic
Quickly	Basic	Pathetic
Skydive	Task	
Blackboard	Stroke	

MOTOR SPEECH

/k/ sentences

1. Kindly keep the kisses for your cutie.
2. I'm calling to confirm your chiropractic consultation.
3. My cousins kept kicking the basketball.
4. The chemical kills the critters that crawl in the cupboard.
5. The cows kept me company in the country.
6. I canned the kernels of corn in the kitchen.
7. The kitten clawed the comfortable couch.
8. I care for the cabbage and carrots quite carefully.
9. Please clear old clay from the corner of the kiln.
10. Quietly, the creature crept through the quiet kingdom.

MOTOR SPEECH

/g/ initial

Go	Gawk	Glacier	Gullible
Goo	Golf	Grammar	Granary
Goal	Green	Gander	Glossary
Good	Gray	Graphite	Godfather
Goof	Grain	Gossip	Gazebo
Gate	Ghost	Glamour	Groveling
Gaze	Glory	Granny	Guaranteed
Gauze	Garbage	Greatness	Glorify
Goat	Given	Gravy	Gardener
Gob	Guitar	Greasy	Gunpowder
Gal	Garden	Galore	Gratefully
Gain	Goodness	Global	Gossiping
Gang	Golden	Gamble	Gravelly
Gone	Glitter	Gravity	Glistening
Goop	Gala	Government	Graciously
Gap	Giver	Graduate	Giveaway
Gore	Grandma	Gallery	Greediness
Gear	Gracious	Gasoline	Greenery
Goes	Guilty	Gratitude	
Got	Greatest	Glorious	
Gross	Gloomy	Groceries	
Gas	Goldfish	Grandmother	

MOTOR SPEECH

/g/ medial & final

Sugar	Snuggle	Vogue
Yogurt	Polygon	Groundhog
Burger	Bigot	Colleague
Forget	Foggy	Monologue
Triangle	Piggy	Vague
Again	Bugle	League
Yoga	Angry	Fatigue
Regular	Leg	Leapfrog
Negative	Rag	Smog
Figure	Blog	Bootleg
Cognition	Drug	Handbag
Jagged	Bag	Jitterbug
Magazine	Debug	Unplug
Pentagon	Unclog	Egg
Jungle	Sheepdog	Shrug
Ergonomics	Flag	Dog
Legal	Prologue	Backlog
Logger	Nutmeg	
Stargaze	Analog	
Flagship	Jetlag	

/g/ sentences

1. Go for the gold though the gamble is great.
2. Goodness gracious, the grandkids are growing.
3. Getting to Grand Central was a gargantuan globetrot.
4. Give us the goods or get gone.
5. The grass grew and the garden was green.
6. The gas in the garage gives off a gross fragrance.
7. Give the gossiping girls a grateful grin.
8. Google grew to global governance.
9. The gala was glistening with golden lights and garlands.
10. The gloomy guesthouse held a gathering of ghosts.

MOTOR SPEECH

/ʃ/ initial

She	Chef	Shoestring	Shortlisted
Shoe	Shut	Shoreline	Shortcoming
Shy	Short	Shorten	Shopkeeper
Shift	Shine	Shocking	Showered
Shell	Shake	Shifty	Shrubbery
Shout	Sharp	Shameless	Shadowy
Show	Shop	Shipwreck	Showering
Shot	Shadow	Sheepskin	Sugary
Shed	Shower	Shape-wear	Shivering
Shape	Shovel	Shackles	Shockingly
Share	Shampoo	Sharpen	Sheepherder
Sheep	Shoelace	Shamrock	Sheepishness
Ship	Sugar	Shipping	Showstopping
Shirt	Shedding	Shrapnel	Shipwrecking
Shark	Shady	Shortcut	Shareholder
Shade	Shiver	Sharpener	Shininess
Sheer	Shopping	Shortsighted	Showboating
Shield	Shoulder	Sharpshooter	Shriveling
Shack	Shatter	Shamelessly	Shadowbox
Shelf	Showman	Shipbuilding	Shutterless
Sham	Shaky	Shuffleboard	Shantytown
Shrimp	Shellfish	Sheepishly	

MOTOR SPEECH

/ʃ/ medial & final

Mushroom	Citizenship	Ambush
Flashlight	Workshop	Banish
Pushup	Vanquishes	Finish
Cashew	Flashback	Blush
Cashier	Fishhooks	Harsh
Marshy	Junkshop	Leash
Action	Squeamishly	Toothbrush
Bushes	Meshwork	Polish
Dishes	Rickshaw	Squash
Fashion	Banshee	Licorice
Ocean	Brush	Eyelash
Machine	Whitewash	Replenish
Lotion	Swordfish	Punish
Tissue	Diminish	Relish
Washer	Foolish	Trash
Emotion	Lush	Mustache
Beneficial	Abolish	Flash
Dictionary	Ash	Tarnish
Bashful	Refresh	Astonish

MOTOR SPEECH

/ʃ/ sentences

1. Surely the shortcut shall show us the finish?
2. I shivered shirtless in the shadows.
3. Shifty men in the shantytown vanished into the shrubs.
4. The chef dished the shallots and shellfish with a flourish.
5. I shun showy shareholders who are selfish and shallow.
6. The shepherd shouted over the shearing of his sheep.
7. Should I shop for the shower shampoo?
8. The shopkeeper and cashier shut down the shop.
9. I showcased the sugary shortbread cookies.
10. He shaved his mustache before the show.

MOTOR SPEECH

/tʃ/ initial

Chow	Chore	Chilly	Charcoal
Chap	Champ	Chipmunk	Cheerios
Chip	Chimp	Chapter	Cheerleader
Cheer	Chomp	Challenge	Cheeseburger
Chase	Choice	Charming	Challenging
Cheat	Chirp	Cheaply	Champion
Chop	Chain	Cheeky	Changeable
Cheese	Chock	Chosen	Chimpanzee
Chair	Chick	Chewing	Chihuahua
Chalk	Chicken	Channel	Chickenpox
Change	Cheetah	Cheaper	Chewing gum
Check	Cherry	Chopsticks	Charmingly
Chin	Children	Cheery	Charity
Cheek	Child	Chestnut	Checkerboard
Chat	Chimney	China	Channeling
Cheap	Chocolate	Chuckle	Chariot
Choose	Checkers	Chapstick	Chickadee

MOTOR SPEECH

/tʃ/ medial & final

Crunchy	Cultural	Ranch
Kitchen	Amateur	Sandwich
Teacher	Merchandise	Sketch
Ketchup	Fetching	Switch
Stitches	Hunchback	Wrench
Pitcher	Hitchhiker	Cockroach
Marches	Sketchbook	Blowtorch
Stretches	Catcher	Stopwatch
Hatching	Rematch	Overreach
Peaches	Spinach	Goldfinch
Statue	Quench	Branch
Reaching	Witch	Latch
Temperature	Couch	Word-search
Achieve	Bench	Stagecoach
Exchange	Impeach	Pouch
Future	Scotch	Preach
Inches	Ostrich	
Question	Pitch	
Touching	Avalanche	
Natural	Scratch	
Signature	Reattach	

/tʃ/ sentences

1. The chattering children were cheering their teacher.
2. Eating cheese and chocolate with chopsticks is challenging.
3. I was chided for chomping the Cheerios.
4. Chuck some charcoal in the chimney on this chilly day.
5. The cheaper China plates chip when chucked.
6. Check the next channel for the chess championship.
7. The chariot charged at the champions.
8. The charming cheerleader chatted with the catcher.
9. The chickadee chirped cheerfully from the chestnut tree.
10. The charity was chock full of chums and chaps.

MOTOR SPEECH

/dʒ/ initial

Judge	Jerk	Judgement	Jubilance
Juice	Jug	Jigsaw	Jeopardy
Just	Jest	Jogger	Jaywalking
Jay	Gel	Jockey	Jackrabbit
Joy	Junk	Jackpot	Joyfulness
Jack	Joust	Jumbled	Juxtapose
June	Jolt	Jitters	Judgmental
Jam	Join	Juggle	Journalist
Jet	Joyous	Jarring	Jamaica
Jar	Journey	Jamming	Jessica
Jade	Justice	Jaunty	Jonathan
Jazz	July	Jaundice	Jovial
Job	Java	Jailer	Jurassic
Jump	Jealous	Gymnast	Justified
Jaw	Jacket	Joystick	Javelin
Jab	Japan	Joyfully	Jamboree
Jeans	Journal	Jealousy	Jawbreaker
Jock	Joker	Jupiter	Jettison
Jail	Jewel	Juniper	Juiciness
Gym	Juicy	Jewelry	Jauntily
Jinx	Jury	Japanese	Journeyman
Juke	Jumping	Jugular	Jarringly

MOTOR SPEECH

/dʒ/ medial & final

Object
Subject
Pajamas
Bejeweled
Injury
Banjos
Bungee
Conjoin
Reject
Injected
Major
Project
Adjust
Ninja
Hijack
Lockjaw
Killjoy
Bluejay
Conjure
Majesty

Enjoyment
Majority
Rejoice
Disjointed
Magic
Infringed
Graduate
Soldier
Teenager
Oranges
Pages
Surgeon
Carriage
Bridge
Stage
Language
Package
Privilege
Challenge
Range

Coverage
Hinge
Emerge
Damage
Wage
Huge
Urge
Submerge
Charge
Offstage
Exchange
Strange
Stooge
Upstage
Advantage
Scavenge
Passage
Mismanage
Disadvantage

MOTOR SPEECH

/dʒ/ sentences

1. Jack and Jill just need a jug of juice.
2. The journalist jeered at the judge's justice.
3. The jailer jabbed the juvenile jauntily.
4. The jock juggled the javelin with joy.
5. Stop jamming the jukebox with junk music.
6. The joker jested and jumped upstage.
7. The Japanese jogger joined a gym.
8. The jams and jellies were injected with oranges.
9. Her jaundice submerges in June and July.
10. The jazz musicians were jamming at the jamboree.

MOTOR SPEECH

/ʒ/ medial & final

Equation
Confusion
Television
Usual
Visual
Measure
Pleasure
Version
Luxury
Decision
Conclusion
Immersion
Diffusion
Corrosion
Diversion
Precision
Unusual
Casual
Foreclosure

Enclosure
Composure
Exposure
Treasure
Leisure
Seizure
Asia
Amnesia
Beige
Camouflage
Collage
Entourage
Garage
Massage
Mirage
Sabotage
Montage

MOTOR SPEECH

/j/ initial

You	Yoke	Yearly	Yellowish
Yes	Yule	Yearning	Yearningly
Yeah	Yield	Yachting	Youthfulness
Yo	Yam	Yielded	Yardmaster
Yawn	Yank	Youngling	Yellowtail
Yin	Yep	Yukon	Yardstick
Yang	Yard	Yeoman	Yeastiness
Yup	Yum	Yiddish	Yesterday
Your	Yikes	Yelping	Youthfully
Y'all	Yonder	Yielding	Yabbering
Yip	Yawning	Yeasty	Yeastiest
Yack	Yodel	Yucky	Yellowfin
Yurt	Yeti	Yawner	Yumminess
Yarn	Yellow	Yahoo	Yarmulke
Yet	Yippee	Yodeling	Yawningly
Year	Yankee	Yosemite	Yesiree
Youth	Yourself	Yellowstone	Yogurt
Yen	Yoga	Yucatan	Yearbooking
Yacht	Yammer	Yakima	
Yeast	Youthful	Yammering	
Yearn	Yummy	Yodeler	

MOTOR SPEECH

/j/ medial

Lawyer	Communion
Loyal	Million
Reuse	Pavilion
Royal	Toyota
Coyote	Unyielding
Reunion	Backyard
Teriyaki	Foyer
Himalaya	Computer
Abuse	Value
Hugely	Canyon
Amusing	Infuse
Confuse	Askew
Misuse	Miscue
Interview	Preview
Review	Rescue

MOTOR SPEECH

/j/ sentences

1. You yearn to return to Yosemite and Yellowstone.
2. I yanked the yellowtail onto the yacht.
3. The yeast yielded a yellowish loaf.
4. Yawning, I ate the yummy yogurt.
5. Yoga will make you more youthful.
6. He yammered about his year in Yakima.
7. The unique yarmulke was made from yarn.
8. The huge Yucatan yams were yellow.
9. The youth lives in a yurt in the Yukon.
10. Ya'll see that Yankee down yonder?

MOTOR SPEECH

/h/ initial

Hot	Have	Hairy	Hamburger
Hope	Hey	Hustle	Happening
Heat	Hi	Homegirl	Helium
Had	Her	Handy	Honeymoon
Hide	Hip	Healthy	Hypocrite
Hog	Heart	Homeless	Hollywood
Hawk	Hard	Hearten	Hibiscus
Hole	Hood	Hopeful	Hazardous
Hill	Hello	Having	Hickory
Him	Human	Heyday	Handkerchief
Home	Happen	Hipster	Hesitant
Ham	Holly	Hoodie	Hairstyle
Honk	Holy	Hippy	Heartwarming
Horn	Happy	Hawkeye	Hideous
Hack	Hungry	Heater	Holistic
Hat	Hollow	Himself	Honeybee
Hair	Humble	History	Hammering
Haste	Hometown	Halloween	Highlighter
Has	Heartless	Homecoming	Halibut
His	Helpful	Hospital	Hangover
Hit	Harmful	Hillbilly	Humdinger
Hatch	Humane	Honkytonk	

MOTOR SPEECH

/h/ medial

Rehearsal	Reheat
Forehead	Overhaul
Inhale	Bellhop
Exhale	Jarhead
Inherit	Overhype
Unhappy	Unharmonious
Inhumane	Fishhook
Backhanded	Keyhole
Dehumidify	Seahawk
Childhood	Blowhole
Blockhead	Withheld
Mohawk	Beehive
Foxhole	Uphill
Bloodhound	Cornhusk
Mishap	Behavior

MOTOR SPEECH

/h/ sentences

1. The hopeful homeowners left their humble hometown.
2. I hear her husband had a heart attack.
3. Please help him hoist the hay bale.
4. The honeybees hummed in harmony.
5. My hair looks horrible and hideous.
6. The harbor is hazardous during a hurricane.
7. The heater helped hearten the homeless.
8. Don't honk the horn near the hospital.
9. I helped myself to heaping hocks of ham.
10. The hooligan held his head up high.

VOICE & RESONANCE

Voice and resonance disorders are problems with the quality, pitch, and/or loudness of the voice. They include difficulties with respiration, phonation, and/or resonance. Choose goals and techniques based on the patient's previous and current levels of functioning, need for referrals, amount of support available, motivation, and other relevant factors.

Voice treatment includes:
- Direct treatment (e.g. specific exercises and techniques to create a healthier voice)
- Indirect treatment (e.g., referral to counseling for stress management and education in vocal hygiene)
- Surgical or pharmacologic intervention (treatment should include any necessary referrals)

Resonance treatment includes:
- Behavioral treatment (e.g. behavioral techniques to improve hypernasality)
- Surgical, prosthetic, or pharmacologic intervention (treatment should include any necessary referrals)

VOICE & RESONANCE

Therapist Instructions

EVALUATIONS. Complete an oral mechanism examination and collect a connected speech sample and reading sample.
- Measure vocal quality using the *Consensus Auditory-Perceptual Evaluation of Voice* available on ASHA.org.
- Complete an acoustic analysis using software such as *Praat* (Boersma, n.d.)
- Complete an aerodynamic assessment, including maximum phonation time, subglottal pressure, and airflow.
- Test resonance using nasal-loaded sentences, nose pinch while reading non-nasal sentences, and the modified tongue anchor test.

DAY ONE OF TREATMENT. Provide the following handouts, as needed:
- Homework Log, Monthly Calendar, Voice & Resonance Impairments, Hypernasality, Nasal Air Emission, Cul-de-Sac Resonance, Vocal Tension, Vocal Weakness, Normal Resonance, Amplification, Vocal Hygiene, GERD Tips
- See the Motor Speech chapter for information about Clear Speech Strategies (page 446), Diaphragmatic Breathing (page 448), and Breath Control (page 450).

FOR THERAPIST EYES ONLY. Pages marked with a gray background or header are resources for therapists. Some caregivers and patients may benefit from having a copy.
- Biofeedback for Voice, Circumlaryngeal Massage

STRATEGIES. Choose 2-3 of the most useful strategies for each patient.
- Hypernasality, Nasal Emission, Cul-de-Sac Resonance, Vocal Tension, Vocal Weakness, Normal Resonance
- Review the selected strategies, provide a model, then ask for return demonstrations. Have these handouts available each session, and refer to them often. Provide caregiver training as needed.

VOICE & RESONANCE

READING MATERIAL. See the Aphasia and Motor Speech chapters for more word lists and for reading material to practice strategies.

TREATING TENSION. Provide the Vocal Tension handout (page 540) to your patient. Consider the following treatment techniques:

- **Stretch-and-Flow** consists of a hierarchy of vocal tasks that balance respiration, phonation, and resonance (Watts et al., 2015). Patients complete increasingly complex tasks (from prolonged exhales to dialogue) using increased muscle activity (from voiceless sighs to normal airflow, speech rate, and fundamental frequency).
- **Resonant Voice Therapy** is used to treat muscle tension dysphonia. The goal of this therapy is to produce a strong, clean voice with the least amount of vocal effort. The patient produces nasal and non-nasal sounds ("meet me Peter meet me"). The clinical manual for this treatment is available for purchase on the publisher's website (Abbott, 2008).
- **Smith Accent Technique** uses controlled breathing and rhythmic exercises to help coordinate vocal fold vibration, air pressure, and air flow (Kotby et al., 1991). The patient begins by producing prolonged voiceless fricatives ("shhh," "ffff," etc.) and gradually produces more complex sounds and eventually conversational speech.

TREATING WEAKNESS. Provide the Vocal Weakness worksheet (page 541) to your patient.

- See Inspiratory Checking, Diaphragmatic Breathing, Breath Control, and Building Up Breath Control (pages 447–452) in the Motor Speech chapter.
- Consider using the following treatment techniques:
  - **Expiratory Muscle Strength Training** (EMST) is for patients with weak coughs and those at risk for aspiration. This includes patients who have Parkinson's disease (Pitts et al., 2009), those weaning from mechanical ventilation, and some post-stroke patients. Training typically involves a specially designed one-way valve (Sapienza & Wheeler, 2006) that only opens and allows airflow when a certain threshold

VOICE & RESONANCE

of effort is reached. EMST devices are available for purchase online *(Aspire, LLC, 2021)*.

- **Lee Silverman Voice Treatment** (LSVT LOUD) was created for people with Parkinson's disease. Its goal is to increase loudness and intelligibility. The program is meant to be intensive, with sessions 4 days a week for 4 weeks. Patients use a loud voice to: produce prolonged, high-pitched, and low-pitched "ah"s; say functional phrases; read aloud; and complete daily homework. Training to become a certified LSVT provider is available online *(LSVT Global, Inc., 2021)*.

- **Vocal Function Exercises** is an exercise regiment that focuses on the use of easy onsets and forward focus in order to increase strength and voice production. The patient produces a prolonged "eee," glides up and down on different words, does tongue and lip trills, and sustains the word "ohl" on different musical notes. Dr. Stemple teaches a vocal function exercise course on MedBridge *(Stemple, n.d.)*

VOICE & RESONANCE

Contents

Biofeedback for Voice	534
Voice & Resonance Impairments	535
Hypernasality	537
Nasal Air Emission	538
Cul-de-Sac Resonance	539
Vocal Tension	540
Vocal Weakness	541
Normal Resonance	542
Amplification	543
Nasal vs. Non-Nasal	544
Easy Onsets	545
Tense Vowels	546
Voiced vs. Voiceless	547
Continuous Voicing	549
Open Vowels	550
Vocal Hygiene	551
Manual Circumlaryngeal Massage	552
Muscles of the Neck Illustration	553
GERD Tips	554

SEE ALSO

Head and Neck Stretches	61
Remembering Reading Material	165
Reading	395
Inspiratory Checking	447
Diaphragmatic Breathing	448
Breath Control	450

VOICE & RESONANCE

Biofeedback for Voice

Biofeedback in the context of voice treatment is the use of sensory feedback (e.g., tactile, auditory, visual) to help patients increase awareness of the physical sensations associated with respiration, resonance, and phonation (ASHA, 2021e). The goal of biofeedback treatment is to improve pitch, loudness, quality, and/or effort.

TACTILE.
- The patient touches their nose to feel vibrations during nasal productions.
- The patient places a hand in front of their nose or mouth during productions to detect airflow.
- The patient places their hands on their chest and stomach to feel diaphragmatic breathing.

AUDITORY.
- Record the patient's voice and play it back to them.
- Place a stethoscope on the patient's nose to detect hypernasality and nasal air emission. If you hear anything through the stethoscope during prolonged non-nasal sounds, that signals hypernasality.

VISUAL.
- Use a sound level meter to measure intensity or loudness.
- Place a tissue or dental mirror under the patient's nose to detect nasal air emission.
- Use a *See-Scape™* device for nasal air emission.
- Use surface electromyography (sEMG) to measure intensity or loudness.

Voice & Resonance Impairments

Common voice and resonance impairments include:

MUSCLE TENSION DYSPHONIA. Makes a strained, weak, high-pitched and/or breathy voice. It is caused by stress, using your voice a lot, laryngopharyngeal reflux, and/or paralyzed vocal folds.

UNILATERAL VOCAL FOLD PARALYSIS. One vocal fold does not move or moves very little. Can cause voice to sound breathy or weak or even cause voicelessness. It is caused by nerve damage from a surgery, stroke, disease, head and neck injury, or a tumor.

BILATERAL VOCAL FOLD PARALYSIS. Both vocal folds do not move. Can cause inspiratory stridor (a noisy, high-pitched sound when breathing in) or voicelessness. It is caused by nerve damage from a surgery, stroke, disease, head and neck injury, or a tumor.

ESSENTIAL VOICE TREMOR. Voice breaks and rhythmic tremors due to involuntary muscle movement. The underlying cause of essential voice tremor is still unknown, though it may be hereditary *(Sulica, 2010)*.

PRESBYLARYNGIS. Age related vocal fold changes. It can cause a softer voice, altered pitch, roughness, and/or vocal tremors.

VOICE & RESONANCE

MYASTHENIA GRAVAS. A condition that can cause hoarseness, vocal fatigue, monotone voice, reduced loudness, inspiratory stridor, and hypernasality *(The Voice Foundation, n.d.)*

HYPOPHONIA. Soft speech. When associated with Parkinson's disease, you may hear reduced vocal loudness (hypokinetic dysarthria), breathy and hoarse voice, and/or tremors.

VOCAL NODULES. Benign bumps on the vocal folds usually related to voice overuse. They can cause a raspy, hoarse, breathy, and easily fatigued voice.

REINKE'S EDEMA. Vocal fold swelling often related to chronic smoking. It can cause a low-pitched and hoarse voice.

HYPERNASALITY. A resonance disorder characterized by too much airflow through the nose while speaking.

NASAL AIR EMISSION. A resonance disorder where excessive airflow is lost out of the nose while speaking.

CUL-DE-SAC RESONANCE. Also known as "potato in the mouth," this is a resonance disorder that causes the voice to sound muffled and almost stuck in the mouth versus resonating out.

VOICE & RESONANCE

Hypernasality

Decrease hypernasality by becoming more aware of it. Learn how to feel and hear when you're being hypernasal.

LISTEN TO & LABEL YOUR VOICE. When you hear yourself being hypernasal, then label it. "I sounded nasally just now."

NASAL vs. ORAL SOUNDS. Say nasal sounds and oral (non-nasal) sounds, such as "ng" (nasal) and "ah" (oral). Notice how they sound different and feel different when you say them.

TACTILE FEEDBACK. Feel the vibrations in the nose when saying nasal sounds, like "nuh," versus non-nasals, like "duh."

WIDE MOUTH OPENING. Over exaggerate your mouth movements while speaking. This increases oral activity (versus nasal activity) and volume *(Kummer, 2008)*.

YAWN/SIGH TECHNIQUE. This is meant to lower back of tongue and raise the velum (the soft back part of the roof of your mouth) to increase oral activity *(Meerschman et al., 2017)*.
1. Pretend that you're going to yawn. Let out a relaxed sigh.
2. While you're sighing, say the following sounds:
   - a, e, i, o, u
   - Maa, paa, baa, faa, vaa, thaw, naw, taw, daw, saw, raw, law
3. Use this technique while speaking throughout the day.

VOICE & RESONANCE

Nasal Air Emission

Decrease nasal air emission by becoming more aware of it. Learn how to feel, hear, and see when air is escaping from your nose while speaking.

AUDITORY FEEDBACK. Record your voice and identify when your resonance is normal versus abnormal. Ask your therapist for help.

TACTILE FEEDBACK. Feel the vibrations in the nose when saying nasal sounds, like "nuh," versus non-nasals, like "duh."

VISUAL FEEDBACK. Place a tissue or dental mirror (available at dollar stores) under your nose and say the following words and sounds. If your resonance is normal, the tissue should not move and the dental mirror should not fog:
- a, e, i, o, u
- Pay, pea, pie, poe, pooh, bay, bee, bye, bow, boo, gay, ghee, guy, go, goo, kay, key, kai, koh, coo, day, dee, die, doh, do, tay, tee, tie, toe, too

NOSE-PINCHING. Pinch your nose while you say the sounds and words above *(NSW Government, 2020)*. Then, un-pinch your nose and say the same sounds. If your resonance is normal, then both sets should sound the same.

VOICE & RESONANCE

Cul-de-Sac Resonance

Decrease cul-de-sac resonance by becoming more aware of it. Learn how to feel and hear when your voice isn't resonating out when it should be.

YAWN-SIGH TECHNIQUE. This is meant to lower back of tongue and raise the velum (the soft back part of the roof of your mouth).

1. Pretend that you're going to yawn. Let out a relaxed sigh.
2. While you're sighing, say the following sounds:
    - a, e, i, o, u
    - Maa, paa, baa, faa, vaa, thaw, naw, taw, daw, saw, raw, law
3. Use this technique while speaking throughout the day.

OPEN MOUTH. Over exaggerate your mouth movements while speaking in order to increase oral activity (versus nasal activity) and volume.

LIP TRILLS. In order to focus your airflow toward the front of your mouth, buzz your lips *(Stemple, n.d.)* Feel the vibration at the front of your face. Try this before speaking so that you remember to project your voice forward.

VOICE & RESONANCE

Vocal Tension

Use the following techniques if you have a tense or tight voice.

CHANT TALK. Read or speak using a monotone, slightly high-pitched voice *(Boone, 1971)*.

YAWN/SIGH TECHNIQUE. This is meant to lower back of tongue and raise the velum (the soft back part of the roof of your mouth).
1. Pretend that you're going to yawn. Let out a relaxed sigh.
2. While you're sighing, say the following sounds:
    - a, e, i, o, u
    - Maa, paa, baa, faa, vaa, thaw, naw, taw, daw, saw, raw, law
3. Use this technique while speaking throughout the day.

CONFIDENTIAL VOICE. Use an easy, breathy, low-airflow voice so that your vocal folds don't completely touch *(Boone, 1971)*.

GLOTTAL FRY. Speak in a low-pitched, creaky, grumbling voice *(Boone, 1971)*.

RELAXATION. Complete stretches (page 61). Ask your therapist for help with massage (page 552).

PRACTICE. Use the following worksheets to practice your vocal tension techniques:
- Easy Onsets, Vowels, Voiced vs. Voiceless, Open Vowels

VOICE & RESONANCE

Vocal Weakness

Use the following techniques if you have a soft or weak voice.

TWANG. Speak using a "twangy" vocal quality, similar to that of a country-western singer (or a witch cackling or a duck quacking!) Adding power to the vocal tract (where the twang is created) will also add power to the voice *(Lombard & Steinhaur, 2007)*.

AMPLIFICATION. See page 543.

BIOFEEDBACK. You can learn to hear and feel vocal weakness. This helps remind you to use a stronger voice.
- Place your hands on your chest and stomach to make sure you're taking deep enough breaths (see Diaphragmatic Breathing on page 448).
- Record your voice and rate your loudness. Many smartphones come preloaded with a voice recording app.
- Use a sound level meter to measure your loudness.

STRENGTHENING PROGRAMS. Speak with your therapist about completing the following treatment programs to strengthen your voice.
- Lee Silverman Voice Treatment
- Vocal Function Exercises
- Expiratory Muscle Strength Training

VOICE & RESONANCE

Normal Resonance

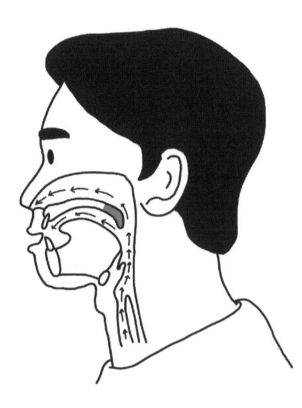

NASAL SOUNDS. For the "m," "n," and "ng" sounds only. The air flows up from the lungs then through the mouth and nose. The velum is relaxed down.

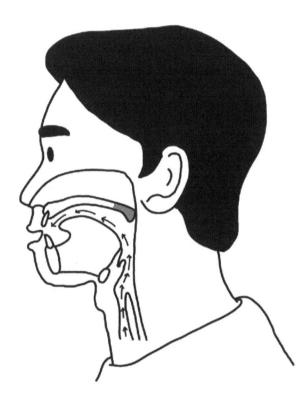

NON-NASAL SOUNDS. For all other sounds. The air flows up from the lungs then through the mouth. The velum rises and blocks off air from entering the nose.

VOICE & RESONANCE

Amplification

Personal amplifiers are available at major retailers, including Amazon.com.

- Amplifiers increase the loudness of your voice in noisy settings, such as at a restaurant or shopping mall.
- Helps avoid yelling and feeling tired after speaking.

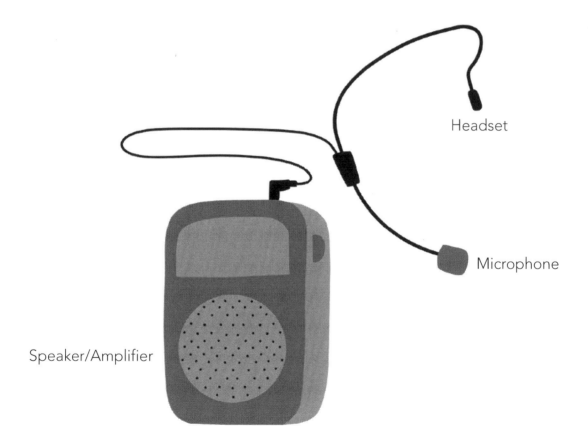

VOICE & RESONANCE

Nasal vs. Non-Nasal

Knowing when you sound nasally can help you achieve normal resonance.

---

1. Close your eyes.

2. Hum the sound "mmmmm" continuously.

3. Gently touch the sides of the bridge of your noise. Feel the vibration.

4. Say "ahhhh" continuously.

5. Gently touch the sides of the bridge of your noise. There should be almost **no** vibration.

6. If you feel a vibration in your nose while saying "ahhh," then use hypernasality tips (see page 537).

VOICE & RESONANCE

Easy Onsets

The following words contain sounds that require a wide, open space in your larynx (voice box). As you read each word aloud, gently move your lips and tongue for easy onsets.

Increase the challenge by ending each word with, "… is the word." For example, "ha is the word."

---

1. Ha
2. How
3. Hoe
4. He
5. Him
6. Who
7. Hash
8. Hole
9. Ham
10. Have
11. Half
12. Hill
13. Hoof
14. Hem
15. Hen
16. Hiss
17. Hail
18. Hair
19. Hall
20. Hear
21. High
22. His

VOICE & RESONANCE

Tense Vowels

These words contain tense vowels (they require more muscle tension to say). Use your voice techniques as your read each word.

Increase the challenge by ending each word with, "… is the word." For example, "Nay is the word."

---

1. Nay
2. Cake
3. Seat
4. Deep
5. Wad
6. Go
7. Mean
8. Raise
9. Take
10. Neat
11. Late
12. Bees
13. Shoe
14. Yeast
15. Spa
16. Loft
17. Day
18. Caught
19. Read
20. Fame
21. Hall
22. Eat
23. Veer
24. Made
25. Leaf
26. Tow
27. Law
28. Sneeze
29. Flee
30. Tree
31. Lease
32. Wage
33. Please
34. Keep

VOICE & RESONANCE

Voiced vs. Voiceless

The words in each word pair differ only by "voicing" (whether or not your vocal folds vibrate). One word starts with a voiced sound, and the other starts with a voiceless sound. Say these words using light contacts: Your lips and tongue should move gently.

Increase the challenge by starting each set with, "The words are … and …."
For example, "The words are gall and call."

---

1. Gall/Call
2. Pass/Bass
3. Pail/Bail
4. Pad/Bad
5. Par/Bar
6. God/Cod
7. Chalk/Jock
8. Tab/Dab
9. Chive/Jive
10. Pig/Big
11. Ped/Bed
12. Peas/Bees
13. Zone/Sown
14. Veer/Fear
15. Zap/Sap
16. Tock/Dock
17. Toll/Dole
18. Tore/Door
19. Jiminey/Chimney
20. Zing/Sing
21. Vaughn/Fawn
22. Gut/Cut
23. Zee/See
24. Poor/Bore
25. Zoo/Sue
26. Gap/Cap

VOICE & RESONANCE

Page 2 of 2

27. Van/Fan
28. Vin/Fin
29. Pun/Bun
30. Veal/Feel
31. Ten/Den
32. Cheese/Jeez
33. Goat/Coat
34. Tell/Dell
35. Zinc/Sink
36. Gob/Cob
37. Tan/Dan
38. Pin/Bin
39. Tow/Doe
40. Tea/Dee
41. Came/Game
42. To/Do
43. Zip/Sip
44. Choke/Joke
45. Peck/Beck
46. Goal/Coal
47. Vee/Fee
48. Till/Dill
49. Pat/Bat
50. Pooh/Boo
51. Zeal/Seal
52. Puck/Buck
53. Tech/Deck
54. Tip/Dip
55. Vat/Fat
56. Pill/Bill
57. Pod/Bod
58. Ton/Done
59. Pam/Bam
60. Peg/Beg
61. Tin/Din
62. Tall/Doll
63. Tear/Dear
64. Pull/Bull
65. Pear/Bear
66. Ted/Dead
67. Gore/Core
68. Gab/Cab

VOICE & RESONANCE

Continuous Voicing

Use your voice techniques while saying the following words. Your vocal folds will vibrate and remain closed while you say each word.

Increase the challenge by ending each word with, "…is the word." For example, "buzz is the word."

---

1. Buzz
2. Dog
3. Road
4. Jam
5. Meal
6. View
7. Bridge
8. Grade
9. Wing
10. Brain
11. Gobble
12. Lemon
13. Jelly
14. Rainbow
15. Yellow
16. Meager
17. Zebra
18. Gravel
19. Driven
20. Ringing
21. Goodbye
22. Thereby
23. Realize
24. Wavering
25. Motherly
26. Remember
27. November
28. Halloween
29. Video
30. Lovingly

VOICE & RESONANCE

Open Vowels

Use your voice techniques while saying the following words. The vowels are "open" which means you need to create a large space in the back of your mouth to say them.

Increase the challenge by ending each word with, "… is the word." For example, "Bomb is the word."

---

1. Bomb
2. Soft
3. Moss
4. Dot
5. Plot
6. Rod
7. All
8. Talk
9. Bat
10. Hat
11. Hot
12. Bath
13. Thought
14. Not
15. Toss
16. Fraud
17. Salt
18. Calm
19. Fought
20. Loft
21. Mom
22. Call
23. Fault
24. Balm
25. Cost
26. Sauce
27. Gone
28. Jog
29. Lull
30. Knot

VOICE & RESONANCE

Vocal Hygiene

The outer layer of the vocal folds are two fragile flaps of tissue that are easy to damage. To avoid vocal fold damage or to heal after damage, follow these guidelines:

WHAT TO DO.

- **Vocal rest.** Give your voice a break! Take "no speaking" breaks throughout the day for 30 minutes at a time (National Institute on Deafness and Other Communication Disorders, 2017).
- **Hydrate.** Drink plenty of water. Water washes away mucus and hydrates the throat. Drink extra water after having alcohol or caffeine.
- **Healthy diet.** Maintaining a healthy diet may contribute to the body's ability to fight off infection and disease. This can improve overall health of the larynx (voice box).

AVOID THE FOLLOWING.

- **Yelling and whispering.** Both increase the risk of damaging the vocal folds.
- **Smoking.** Smoke may irritate and damage the lungs and the vocal folds. Smoking can also induce throat-clearing and coughing, which can damage the vocal folds.
- **Alcohol & caffeine.** Dehydrates the throat. If you do drink alcohol or caffeine, then compensate by drinking an extra cup of water.
- **Coughing & throat clearing.** Too much can irritate and damage the vocal folds.

VOICE & RESONANCE

Circumlaryngeal Massage

Manual circumlaryngeal massage is used to treat muscle tension dysphonia. It aims to lower the larynx into a more neutral position (Roy & Leeper, 1993; ASHA, 2020d). *If your patient continues to experience muscle tension despite massage, consider a mental health referral. Unmanaged stress and other emotional or psychological causes can also result in muscle tension.*

1. Find the thyroid notch with your index finger.
2. Gently run your index finger and thumb laterally until you find the thyroid laminae.
3. Work your fingers superiorly until you locate the hyoid bone.
4. Massage the hyoid using your index finger and thumb, working anterior to posterior until you reach the major cornu. Have the patient hum while you massage. Note any changes in voice.
    - The carotid artery is located close to this area; make sure that you are massaging the hyoid bone and not the artery!
5. Run your fingers inferiorly and medially to the thyroid cartilage and massage the thyroid cartilage using your index finger and thumb. Massage anterior to posterior until you reach the posterior borders of the thyroid cartilage. Have the patient hum while you massage to detect any voice changes, including reduced tension.

VOICE & RESONANCE

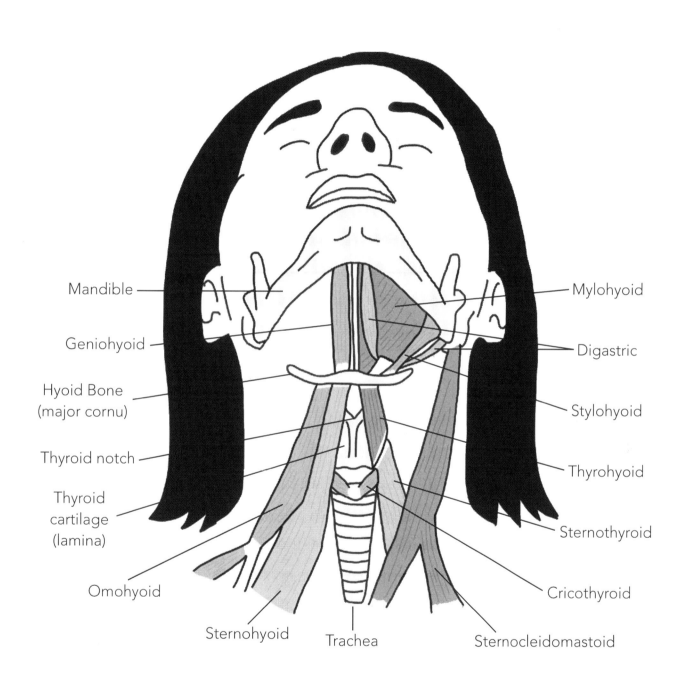

> **VOICE & RESONANCE**

GERD Tips

Gastroesophageal Reflux (GERD or acid reflux) can be managed with the help of the following tips.

- Drink plenty of water
- Sit upright during and after you eat or drink *(Harvard Health Publishing, 2019)*
- Wear loose-fitting clothes around your waist—avoid tight belts and waistbands *(Mayo Clinic Staff, 2020)*
- Eat smaller meals more frequently
    - *For example, eat 5 small meals plus snacks versus 3 large meals*
- Sleep with the head of your bed raised at least 30-45 degrees
    - *For example, use 3 or more pillows while lying in bed*
- Maintain a healthy weight
- Ask your doctor about medications to help manage symptoms
- Avoid caffeinated beverages, including coffee, tea, and soda
- Avoid trigger foods, including tomatoes and citrus fruits
- Avoid fried foods
- Avoid alcohol
- Quit smoking

AUGMENTATIVE & ALTERNATIVE COMMUNICATION

Augmentative and alternative communication (AAC) are methods of communicating besides talking. AAC can be used for patients with cognitive, communication, and/or motor deficits. The goal of AAC treatment is to increase the patient's ability to communicate wants and needs. Choose goals and techniques based on the patient's previous and current levels of functioning, nature of the disease/disability (e.g., acute or progressive), amount of support available, motivation, and other relevant factors.

AAC treatment includes:
- Training in the use of devices
- Incorporating device use in everyday life
- Training facilitators to use the device and support the patient

Therapist Instructions

EVALUATIONS. Choose evaluations based on your patient's disorder or disease. You may evaluate language, cognition, motor speech, vision, hearing, and/or overall physical functioning (e.g., ability to write or type on a keyboard). Refer out to specialists as needed.
- Basics of an AAC evaluation *(Brewer, 2019)*:
    - Complete a case history and support system interview
    - Determine speech rate, intelligibility, language expression and comprehension, and motor abilities
    - Trial AAC devices
    - Identify patient's support system (these people often become the facilitators)
    - Identify what vocabulary needs to be added to the device based on the patient's current needs
    - Add and organize messages on the device and train facilitators
    - Train the patient in other modalities
- Evaluations by diagnosis:
    - For patients with ALS and Parkinson's, start with a motor speech evaluation.
    - For patients with aphasia, start with a language evaluation.
    - Other patients needing AAC may have long-term intubation, myasthenia gravis, head and neck cancer, Guillain-Barre syndrome, etc. Select the most appropriate evaluation for each patient.

DAY ONE OF TREATMENT. Provide the following handouts, as needed:
- Homework Log, Monthly Calendar, What is AAC, AAC Ideas, Listener Tips, Alphabet Board, Needs Board

FOR THERAPIST EYES ONLY. The Device Trials (page 559) is marked with a gray background and is a resource for therapists.

AAC

CAREGIVER TRAINING. Educate the family and medical team about the basics of your patient's AAC techniques and how to be an effective listener (see page 564).
- Identify a facilitator who will be your patient's primary AAC support at home. This person will receive extensive training in the AAC and communication needs of your patient.
- Involve other close family members and friends by asking for input on meaningful messages to add (e.g. a fishing buddy can recommend fishing-related words). Educate on AAC communication strategies.

TRANSIENT AAC USERS. Some patients may only use no-tech or low-tech AAC for a short while. Even if temporary, it's still important to help your patients find an effective, consistent way to communicate as soon as possible.

COMMUNICATION BOARDS. The messages included on the Needs and Code Boards are frequent patient requests. That said, your patients will have their own unique needs and messages. Copy the pertinent boards, fill in the blanks as needed, then place in protective plastic sheets for durability.

PERSONALIZING AAC. This will depend on the patient's wants, needs, likes, dislikes, personality, social life, hobbies, career, etc. Your evaluation will provide this information.
- Add messages as needed; personalizing AAC is a dynamic process.
- Remove messages as needed; some preloaded messages may be irrelevant to your patient.

GOALS. The patient's underlying condition will guide AAC goals. In general, goals include increasing complexity of messages, initiation of use, speed and carryover of use in different communication settings, and caregiver training.

AAC

Contents

Device Trials	559
What is AAC?	561
AAC Ideas	562
Listener Tips	564
Eye Transfer Board	565
E-Tran Board Example	567
Alphabet Board *(instructions)*	568
Alphabet Board	569
Needs Board	570
Code Board	571

AAC

Device Trials

Your patient will likely trial a few devices before finding the right fit. Thankfully, high-tech device manufacturers including Lingraphica® and Tobii Dynavox® offer free device trials so your patient can try a device before purchasing it.

WHY TRIAL DEVICES? A high-tech speech-generating device may be your patient's voice for years. Whether it's a good match depends on your patient's strengths, weaknesses, likes, and dislikes, among other factors. It is also a large financial investment. Therefore, it's best practice to trial a few devices before your patient commits their time and money.

AVAILABLE DEVICES. Research available devices online. Review the specifications to determine which devices match your patient's needs.

COST. Always clarify how much money your patient is willing and able to pay for a device before trials. Speech-generating devices are considered durable medical equipment and are covered in part by Medicare, Medicaid, and some private insurance companies.

HOW TO CHOOSE A DEVICE TO TRIAL. This will be a collaborative process between you, your patient, and their facilitator. Once you identify a few promising devices, print out information for your patient. Share videos of the devices being used. Discuss which devices seems like the best fit.

STARTING A TRIAL. Contact the company online or by phone. Representatives are typically prompt, helpful, and forthcoming.

AAC

QUESTIONS FOR THE COMPANY. Get the most out of your call with the representative by having a list of questions ready. Ask about cost, length of trials, how to return a device, who to call for technical help, etc.

INSURANCE COVERAGE. Companies may require the patient's insurance information prior to lending a device. Ask the representative for step-by-step instructions on how to submit this information.

PATIENT TRIALS. Once the device arrives, complete a preliminary personalization of the device by adding and deleting messages based on your patient's wants and needs.
- Review the device with your patient. Show them the overall layout and organization. Model how to type, create phrases and sentences, add and delete vocabulary, and change settings.
- Complete a device trial evaluation. This will be similar to a communication evaluation. Ask the patient to:
  - Locate icons, match icons to words, type words, phrases, and sentences; build phrases and sentences using icons; and participate in conversation.
  - Provide cues and prompts as needed to increase accuracy and avoid frustration.

INCLUDE THE FACILITATORS. The patient's preferences, wants, and needs are your top priority. However, facilitator feedback and training is also important for AAC to be successful.

IDENTIFYING A "GOOD MATCH."
- The patient can communicate their wants and needs using the device.
- The patient navigates the device with minimal to no frustration.
- During the trial period, the patient shows some progress in speed and/or complexity of messages produced.
- The patient can afford the device.

AAC

What is AAC?

Augmentative & Alternative Communication (AAC) includes all the ways to communicate without talking.

- Most of us use AAC everyday—we make hand gestures, nod our heads, point, make facial expressions, write, and text.

- The purpose of AAC is to give people a reliable way to effectively communicate their wants and needs in ways other than talking.

- AAC isn't necessarily meant to replace talking but rather to supplement or support talking.

- The amount and type of AAC people need depends on their communication strengths and weakness, physical abilities, and likes and dislikes.

- Speech therapists are experts in communication, whether it be talking or using AAC.

AAC Ideas

NO-TECH AAC. Communicating without specialized technology.
- Writing with felt-tip pens and a notepad
    - If possible, opt for felt-tip pens. They're easier for patients to write with and result in less accidental marks.
- Writing with a dry-erase marker and a whiteboard
- Writing using a magic slate or *Buddha Board™*
- Nodding, shaking head, shrugging
- Pointing, nodding head to the right or left
- Finger spelling (e.g. tracing letters in the air or on a table)

LOW-TECH AAC. Communicating with everyday technology.
- Texting with a phone or tablet
- Using a communication board
- Using a plexiglass or Eye Transfer board (page 565)
- Using an alphabet board (page 569)
- Using a needs board (page 570)
- Using a code board (page 571)
- Typing on a computer or laptop
- Using text-to-speech apps or narrator programs on computers
- Using a tablet (preferably 10" wide or larger)
    - *iPad Pro®, Microsoft® Surface*

HIGH-TECH AAC. Communicating with specialized technology.
- Speech-generating devices
    - Tobii DynaVox, Lingraphica
- AAC apps on tablets
    - *Proloquo2go™, LetMeTalk*

ALTERNATIVE ACCESS. AAC for patients with limited use of their hands.
- Styluses or laser pointers to point to items on communication boards or tablets
- Switches and joysticks to scan and select items on high-tech systems
    - *AbleNet®, Smartnav™, Enabling Devices, School Health®*
- Trackballs and touch-pads to navigate high-tech systems
    - School Health, AbleNet
- Head tracking and eye gaze to navigate high-tech systems
    - Tobii, *PRC-Saltillo, Eyegaze, Inc.*

> AAC

Listener Tips

Use the following tips to help you successfully start and continue a conversation with someone using an AAC device. The flow of conversation is different from talking, so be prepared for longer pauses.

- Have the conversation in a quiet setting
- Reduce distractions: turn off the TV, silence your cellphone, etc.
- Make eye contact often and avoid staring at the AAC screen
- Speak directly to the person and not the assistant or caregiver
- Ask open-ended questions (**not** yes or no questions) to encourage conversation *(Communication Matters, n.d.)*
- Wait at least 5 seconds for each response
- If you're feeling lost in the conversation:
    - Be honest if you're having a hard time understanding
    - Continue speaking directly to the person while making eye contact
    - Confirm what you think you understood by repeating it back to them
    - Ask to confirm the subject. "Are we still discussing…?"
    - If either of you start feeling frustrated, then move on to the next subject and come back to it later

| AAC |

Eye Transfer Board

An E-Tran board allows your patient to communicate via eye gaze. It consists of six large boxes containing six letters/numbers with a repeating color system. See the model on page 567. For an example in full color, see Ace Centre's E-tran website.

MAKING THE BOARD.

1. Copying the model on page 567, type the text of each box into 6 separate word documents. Use text size 36 or larger. Print using **color** ink.
    - Make **each letter/number** the correct color *(Ace Centre, 2021)*. From left to right: green (top left of each box), yellow, black, gray (bottom left of each box), blue, red.
    - Outline **each box** with the correct color. You will cut them out and place them in this order on the board. From left to right: green (top left box), yellow, black, gray (bottom left box), blue, red.
2. Adhere the papers to a large (at least 18" wide) piece of plexi-glass (durable, easy to clean) or foam board (cheap, easy to work with).
    - For foam boards, cut out a large rectangle in the middle of the board so you can see the patient's eyes.

REFERENCE BOARD. Print out a small, mirror-image version of the E-Tran board (see page 567).

- The numbers and letters will be the same colors as the patient's board, but the layout will be a mirror image.
- You will use the reference board to check which letter/number the patient is gazing at.

USING A BOARD.
- Place yourself eye-to-eye with the patient. Hold the E-Tran board up to your eye-level. Watch their eyes.
- Ask the patient to spell their message using the following technique:
  1. Ask them to gaze at the box that **contains the first target letter/number**. Check your reference board, then say the color of the main box to confirm.
  2. Next, ask them to gaze at the box that is **outlined by the same color** that the **target letter/number is colored**. Say the color of the second box to confirm.
  3. You can now state the target letter/number.

To summarize, the patient spells out messages by gazing at different-colored boxes. Confirm each box color, then confirm the target letter/number. **Each letter/number requires 2 gazes to "select."**
- *Example: Spelling out "TV"*
- *The patient gazes at the gray outlined main box, then the red outlined main box to select "T"*
- *The patient gazes at the blue outlined main box, then the blue outlined main box again to select "V"*

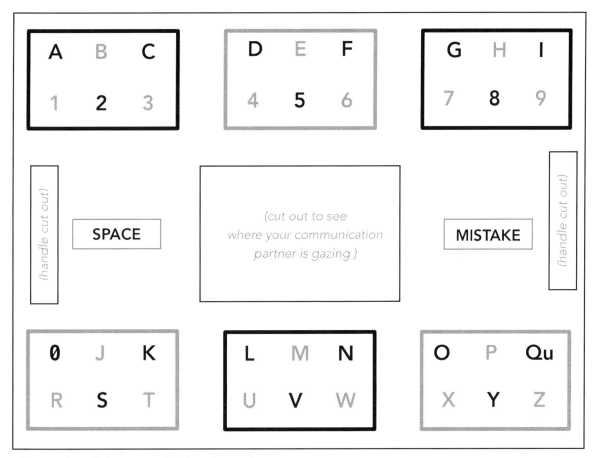

Example of the main E-Tran board.

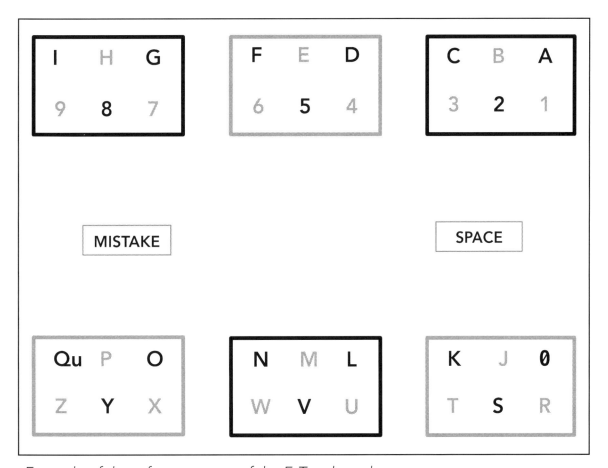

Example of the reference copy of the E-Tran board.

AAC

Alphabet Board

A simple alphabet board can help a person communicate their wants and needs. Make a copy then keep it in a protective plastic sleeve.

WAYS TO USE AN ALPHABET BOARD.
- The patient points to the first letter of the word and says the word.
- The patient spells out the entire word.
- The patient spells out the code for a message on their code board (see page 571).

TIPS FOR THE LISTENER.
- Make sure that the alphabet board is always within the patient's reach.
- Give the patient plenty of time to select each letter.
- Confirm each letter the patient chooses by saying it aloud.
- Only guess a word when you're 90% sure you know what the word is.

```
A  B  C  D  E  F  G
H  I  J  K  L  M  N
O  P  Q  R  S  T  U
V  W  X  Y  Z
1  2  3  4  5  6  7  8  9  0   YES  NO
```

Medicine	Food	Drink	Thank you	I love you!
Toilet	Toothbrush	Bed	Suction	Tissue
Pain	Head up	Head down	T.V.	Telephone
				OTHER

AAC

Code Board

If your main form of communication is typing or writing, then use this Code Board to reduce the amount of time needed to select common messages. For example, instead of selecting "t, h, a, n, k, y, o, u," you can type "t y" to indicate "Thank you." Add your own messages as needed.

TY	Thank you.
UN	Can you adjust my position? I'm uncomfortable.
PA	I have some pain.
PI	Can you move my pillows?
BA	I need to use the bathroom.
GN	Good night.
LY	I love you.
MD	May I have my medicine?
____	_____
____	_____
____	_____
____	_____
____	_____
____	_____

FLUENCY

A fluency disorder is a disruption to smooth, forward-flowing speech. The goal of fluency treatment is to reduce the severity of disfluencies. Choose goals and techniques based on the patient's previous and current levels of functioning, nature of the disorder (e.g., neurological, psychological, etc.), motivation, and other relevant factors.

Fluency treatment includes:
- Speech modification (e.g., prolonged speech and easy onsets)
- Stuttering modification (e.g., cancellations and pull outs)
- Reducing the negative impact a fluency disorder has on a patient's life (e.g., desensitization and cognitive restructuring). See asha.org for more information.

FLUENCY

Therapist Instructions

EVALUATIONS. Collect a case history, conversational speech sample, reading sample, and five-minute monologue.
- Complete a molecular analysis using the five-minute monologue speech sample to determine percent of stuttering disfluencies and percent normal disfluencies.
- Complete a norm-referenced evaluation such as the *Stuttering Severity Instrument* (approximately 20 minutes to complete) and a questionnaire such as the *Locus of Control Behaviour* scale.

DAY ONE OF TREATMENT. Provide the following handouts, as needed:
- Homework Log, Monthly Calendar, Fluency Impairments, Fluency Strategies, Anatomy & Physiology, Breath Curve

STRATEGIES. Review the fluency strategies and breath curve, provide a model, then ask for return demonstrations. Review the strategies often.

FOR THERAPIST EYES ONLY. The Treatment Techniques page (576) has a gray background and is a resource for therapists.

ANATOMY & PHYSIOLOGY (PAGE 580). Review this worksheet with your patient before beginning treatment. Improved body awareness can make treatment more effective.

READING MATERIAL. Start with Light vs. Hard Sounds (page 582) to practice the fluency strategies.
- Use the phonemic lists in the Motor Speech chapter (page 464) for additional words.
- Advance to longer reading material from other chapters to practice fluency strategies.

FLUENCY

Contents

Treatment Techniques	576
Fluency Impairments	578
Fluency Strategies	579
Anatomy & Physiology	580
Breath Curve	581
Light vs. Hard Sounds	582

Treatment Techniques

Ask the patient to first practice these techniques while reading aloud. Gradually work towards using them in conversation (see pages 358–360 and 455 for conversation topics).

REDUCED SPEECH RATE. The patient starts by producing about 1 syllable per second, stretching out each sound. Insert pauses between words and syllables (Logan, n.d.)
- Read aloud in unison with your patient, using a slow rate.
- Slowly fade out the amount you read aloud in unison.
- Eventually model reading aloud at a slow rate, then ask the patient to copy you.

PROLONGED SPEECH. Also known as smooth speech, this is a fluency shaping technique. It reduces speech rate and stuttering behaviors by prolonging syllables. The patient is gradually trained to speak at a normal rate (Logan, n.d.)
- "Heee leeeaves ooon Friiidaaay."

BREATH CURVE (PAGE 581). The breath curve is a simple image that helps patients visualize how to coordinate respiration with phonation.
- The patient is asked to take a full breath then phonate shortly after exhalation begins (Hogan, 2004). They may use this while reading or speaking.

EASY ONSETS. Avoid hard vocal attacks by using /h/. This is a phoneme that allows for maximum, easy airflow.
- Ask the patient to begin by producing /h/ plus a vowel sound. Follow with /h/ initial words (page 526), /h/ initial sentences, then phrases that begin with vowel sounds.

LIGHT ARTICULATORY CONTACTS. The articulators move and touch gently. To reduce articulatory tension, teach your patient the difference between a hard versus light contact.
- For instance, teach the difference between producing /h/ and /p/. Ask the patient to complete the contrast drills on page 582 while using light contacts (Kuster, n.d.)

FLUENCY

CONTINUOUS VOICING AND AIRFLOW. Ask the patient to "keep the motor going" by saying the entire production or sentence without any breaks (until they need to take a breath; ASHA, 2021a).

CANCELLATIONS. Teach the patient to first pause for a few seconds after stuttering and then say the word again with less tension.
- "F-f-f- [pause]. Ffffriday."

PULL OUTS. When a patient stutters, ask them to pull or slide out of it as they continue voicing to avoid a stoppage or block.
- "H-h-h- [slide out] hhhhhe leaves on Friday."

PREPARATORY SETS. When a patient anticipates that they will stutter on a sound, ask them to "ease" into the word by slightly prolonging the initial sound.
- "He [ease into it] llleaves on Friday."

METRONOME. Help your patient self-pace and speak at a slower rate by using a metronome (Brady, 1971).
- Prompt the patient to produce one syllable or word per beat, gradually increasing the speed to a normal speaking rate.

CHORAL SPEECH. Read aloud in unison with your patient, fading out until the patient is reading aloud alone (Kalinowski & Saltuklaroglu, 2003).

SHADOWING. The patient reads from a script in unison with a recording of the same script (A-Rong-Na & Sakai, 2015).

PACING. Write out target words or phrases for your patient and place a dot under each syllable.
- Ask your patient to touch each dot and produce one syllable per dot.
- Continuing the pace of one dot per syllable, gradually introduce phase completions then sentences (Gully, 2018).

Fluency Impairments

Common fluency impairments include:

NEUROGENIC STUTTERING. Stuttering caused by brain damage, most commonly a stroke.

PHARMACOGENIC STUTTERING. Stuttering caused by medication side-effects. Talk to your doctor and pharmacist to address this type of stuttering.

PSYCHOGENIC STUTTERING. Stuttering caused by psychological or emotional issues (but not malingering). Seek out therapy or psychiatric services to address this type of stuttering.

DEVELOPMENTAL STUTTERING. The most common form of stuttering. When the stutter develops in childhood.

FLUENCY

Fluency Strategies

- Relax your body and take a full breath
- Begin speaking shortly after exhaling
- Use easy onsets—your vocal folds should touch gently *(Molt & Yaruss, 2021)*
- Use light contacts—your mouth and tongue should touch gently
- Slow down and stretch out the sounds
- If you stutter, pause for a few seconds then say it again.

FLUENCY

Anatomy & Physiology

To speak, you must coordinate breathing, making sounds, and shaping sounds. Stuttering can happen when any of these are interrupted.

RESPIRATION. Breathing for speech.
- You breathe in, your vocal folds open, and your lungs expand and fill with air.
- You breathe out, air rushes out from your lungs and between your vocal folds.

PHONATION. Creating sounds.
- Just before you speak, you exhale and your vocal folds close.
- Sound is created when air rushes through your closed vocal folds.

ARTICULATION. Shaping sounds into speech.
- The sound created by your vocal folds travels up your throat and out of your mouth and/or nose.
- You move your tongue, lips, jaw, and palate (back of the roof of the mouth) to shape all the speech sounds.

FLUENCY

Breath Curve

1. Trace the curve with your finger.
2. Inhale on the up-curve.
3. Exhale on the down-curve.
4. Say "haaa" shortly after exhalation begins.
5. Gradually say longer words and sentences whenever your finger traces over the "speak" line.

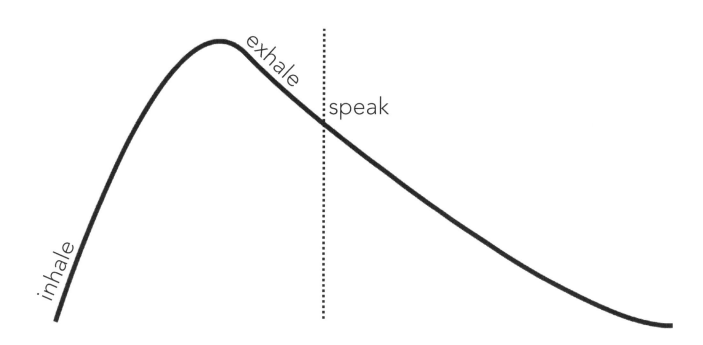

FLUENCY

Light vs. Hard Sounds

Practice using light contacts with both light ("h") versus hard ("p") sounds.

Ha/Pa	Hug/Pug	Hang/Pang
How/Pow	Ham/Pam	Host/Post
Hoe/Poe	Hop/Pop	Heat/Peat
He/Pea	Heal/Peel	Hitch/Pitch
Hi/Pie	Hocus/Pocus	Hair/Pair
Who/Pooh	Hill/Pill	Holly/Polly
Hey/Pay	Hen/Pen	Huddle/Puddle
Hall/Paul	Hut/Putt	Hail/Pail
Hose/Pose	Hack/Pack	Hacked/Pact
Hot/Pot	Hide/Pride	Haste/Paste
Hole/Pole	Hike/Pike	Hearty/Party
Hear/Peer	Hurl/Pearl	Hacking/Packing

References

1. Abbott, K.V. (2008). *Lessac-Madsen Resonant Voice Therapy* [DVD]. San Diego, CA: Plural Publishing, Inc.
2. Abel, S., Schultz, A., Radermarcher, I., Willmes, K., & Huber, W. (2005). Decreasing and increasing cues in naming therapy for aphasia. *Aphasiology, 19*(9), 831-848. DOI: 10.1080/02687030500268902
3. Ace Centre. (2021). *Resources*. Retrieved from https://acecentre.org.uk/resources/
4. American Dental Association. (2019). *Aging and Dental Health*. Retrieved from https://www.ada.org/en/member-center/oral-health-topics/aging-and-dental-health
5. American Heart Association. (2015). *Let's talk about: Complication After Stroke* [Data File]. Retrieved from https://www.stroke.org/-/media/stroke-files/lets-talk-about-stroke/life-after-stroke/ltas_complications-after-stroke.pdf?la=en
6. The American Occupational Therapy Association. (2013). *Living With Low Vision* [Data File]. Retrieved from https://www.aota.org/~/media/Corporate/Files/AboutOT/consumers/Adults/LowVision/Low%20Vision%20Tip%20Sheet.ashx
7. American Speech-Language-Hearing Association. (2021a). *Fluency Disorders*. Retrieved from https://www.asha.org/practice-portal/clinical-topics/fluency-disorders/#collapse_6
8. American Speech-Language-Hearing Association. (2021b). *Dysarthria*. Retrieved from https://www.asha.org/public/speech/disorders/dysarthria/#tips
9. American Speech-Language-Hearing Association. (2021c). *International Classification of Functioning, Disability, and Health (ICF)*. Retrieved from https://www.asha.org/slp/icf/
10. American Speech-Language-Hearing Association. (2021d). *Language/Cognitive-Communication Evaluation* [Data file]. Retrieved from https://www.asha.org/uploadedFiles/AATLanguageCognition.pdf
11. American Speech-Language-Hearing Association. (2021e). *Voice Disorders*. Retrieved from https://www.asha.org/practice-portal/clinical-topics/voice-disorders/#collapse_6
12. Anderson, J. E. (2017). Treatment of Underlying forms and constraint induced auditory training in aphasia: a single case study. *Culminating projects in communication sciences and disorders*, 5.
13. Aparo, M. & Brewer, C.H. (2020). *The Adult Speech Therapy Workbook*. Retrieved from https://www.theadultspeechtherapyworkbook.com/
14. A-Rong-Na, N., & Sakai, K.M. (2015). Short-Term Effects of Speech Shadowing Training on Stuttering. *The Japan Journal of Logopedics and Phoniatrics, 55*(4), 326-334.
15. Aspire, LLC. (2021). *Health & Medical*. Retrieved from https://emst150.com/health-and-medical/
16. Axelrod, J. (2016). *Strategies for Improving Memory*. Retrieved from https://psychcentral.com/lib/strategies-for-improving-memory#1
17. Banks, L. (2020). *6 Ways To Easily Tell If Your Hearing Aid Is On*. Retrieved from https://www.clearliving.com/hearing/hearing-aids/on-off-settings/
18. Barclay, R. (2020). *What Is Hemianopsia?* Healthline Media. Retrieved from https://www.healthline.com/symptom/loss-of-vision-in-one-half-of-the-visual-field
19. Berkley, C. (2006). *Is Your Memory Normal?* WebMD LLC. Retrieved from https://www.webmd.com/alzheimers/features/is-your-memory-normal#1
20. Beurskens, C.H.G., Devriese, P.P., Van Heinigen, I., & Oostendorp, R.A.B. (2004). The use of mime therapy as a rehabilitation method for patients with facial nerve paresis. *International Journal of Therapy and Rehabilitation, 11*(5), 206-210.
21. Beurskens, C.H.G., & Heymans, P.G. (2006). Mime therapy improves facial symmetry in people with long term facial nerve paresis: A randomised controlled trial. *Australian Physiotherapy Association, 52*, 177-183.
22. Bislick L.P., Weir, P.C., Spencer, K., Kendall, D., & Yorkston, K.M. (2012). Do principles of motor learning enhance retention and transfer of speech skills? A systematic review. *Aphasiology, 26*(5), 709-728.
23. Blake, M., Novak, K., & Freer, J. (2016). *Treatment Strategies for Unilateral Visuospatial Neglect and Anosognosia*. Retrieved from https://www.medbridgeeducation.com/blog/2016/02/treatment-strategies-for-unilateral-neglect-and-anosognosia/
24. Boden, K., Hallgren, A., & Witt Hedstrom, H. (2006). Effects of three different swallow maneuvers analyzed by videomanometry. *Acta Radiologica, 47*, 628-633.
25. Boersma, P. [n.d.] *Praat: Doing phonetics by computer*. Retrieved from www.fon.hum.uva.nl/praat

26. Boone, D.R. (1971). *The Voice and Voice Therapy.* Englewood, N.J.: Prentice-Hall.
27. Brady, J.P. (1971). Metronome-conditioned speech retraining for stuttering. *Behavior Therapy, 2*(2), 129-150.
28. Brewer, C.H. (2019). *The Home Health SLP Handbook* (M. Aparo, Ed.). Harmony Road Design, LLC.
29. Brunt, L.M., Eagon, J.C., & Awad, M. [n.d.] *Esophageal Soft Diet* [Data file]. Washington University in St. Louis School of Medicine. Retrieved from https://cpb-us-w2.wpmucdn.com/sites.wustl.edu/dist/0/1329/files/2013/03/Esoph-soft-diet-pamphlet-2-21-2014-1yv96s4.pdf
30. Butler, D.P. & Grobbelaar, A.O. (2017). Facial palsy: what can the multidisciplinary team do? *Journal of Multidisciplinary Healthcare, 10,* 377-381.
31. Caparroz, F.A., Campanholo, M.D.T., Sguillar, D.A., Haddad, L., Park, S.W., Bittencourt, L., Tufik, S., & Haddad, F.L.M. (2019). A Pilot Study on the Efficacy of Continuous Positive Airway Pressure on the Manifestations of Dysphagia in Patients with Obstructive Sleep Apnea. *Dysphagia, 34,* 333-340.
32. Cedars-Sinai. (2021). *Aspiration from Dysphagia.* Retrieved from https://www.cedars-sinai.org/health-library/diseases-and-conditions/a/aspiration-from-dysphagia.html
33. Centers for Disease Control and Prevention. (2020). *Deaths from Older Adult Falls.* Retrieved from https://www.cdc.gov/homeandrecreationalsafety/falls/fallcost/deaths-from-falls.html
34. Chen, P., Hreha, K., Fortis, P., Goedert, K., & Barrett, A. (2012). Functional Assessment of Spatial Neglect: A Review of the Catherine Bergego Scale and an Introduction of the Kessler Foundation Neglect Assessment Process. *Topics in Stroke Rehabilitation, 19*(5), 423-435.
35. Clark, H.M., O'Brien, K., Calleja, A., Corrie, S.N. (2009). Effects of Directional Exercise on Lingual Strength. *Journal of Speech, Language, and Hearing Research, 52,* 1034-1047.
36. Cleveland Clinic. (2019). *Why Improving Your Concentration Helps Your Memory.* Retrieved from https://health.clevelandclinic.org/why-improving-your-concentration-helps-your-memory/
37. Communication Matters. [n.d.] *What is AAC?* Retrieved from https://communicationmatters.org.uk/overview/
38. Cowan, N. (2010). The Magical Mystery Four: How is Working Memory Capacity Limited, and Why?. *Current directions in psychological science, 19*(1), 51–57. https://doi.org/10.1177/0963721409359277
39. Davis, L. A., & Stanton, S. T. (2005). Semantic Feature Analysis as a Functional Therapy Tool. *Contemporary Issues in Communication Science and Disorders, 32,* 85-92.
40. Dawson, D.R., Gaya, A., Hunt, A., Levine, B., Lemsky, C., & Polatajko, H.J. (2009). Using the Cognitive Orientation to Occupational Performance (CO-OP) with adults with executive dysfunction following traumatic brain injury. *Canadian Journal Of Occupational Therapy, 76*(2), 115-127.
41. The Department of Homeland Security. (2021). *Make a Plan.* Retrieved from https://www.ready.gov/plan
42. Donzelli, J., & Brady, S. (2004). The effects of breath-holding on vocal fold adduction: Implications for safe swallowing. *Archives of Otolaryngology–Head & Neck Surgery, 130,* 208–210.
43. Dressler, R.A. (2005). *LARK-2: Language Activity Resource Kit - Second Edition.* Austin, TX: ProEd, Inc.
44. Dysphagia Ramblings. (2019). *Pudding and a straw.* Retrieved from https://dysphagiaramblings.net/2019/10/14/pudding-and-a-straw/
45. Edmonds, L. A., Nadeau, S. E., & Kiran, S. (2009). Effect of Verb Network Strengthening Treatment (VNeST) on Lexical Retrieval of Content Words in Sentences in Persons with Aphasia. *Aphasiology, 3*(3): 402-404.
46. Elfrink, T.R., Zuidema, S.U., Kunz, M., & Westerhof, G.J. (2018). Life story books for people with dementia: a systematic review. *International Psychogeriatrics, 20*(12), 1797-1811. DOI: https://doi.org/10.1017/S1041610218000376
47. Ehlhardt, L.A., Sohlberg, M.M., Glang, A., & Albin, R. (2005). TEACH-M: A pilot study evaluating an instructional sequence for persons with impaired memory and executive functions. *Brain Injury, 19*(8), 569-83.
48. Freutel, N. (2020). *Neck Exercises and Stretches for a Herniated Disc.* Healthline Media. Retrieved from https://www.healthline.com/health/fitness-exercise/herniated-disk-exercises
49. Fujiu, M., & Logemann, J.A. (1996). Effect of a tongue-holding maneuver on posterior pharyngeal wall movement during deglutition. *American Journal of Speech Language Pathology, 5,* 23-30.
50. Gotter, A. (2020). *Box Breathing.* Retrieved from https://www.healthline.com/health/box-breathing
51. Grattan, E.S., & Woodbury, M.L. (2017). Do Neglect Assessments Detect Neglect Differently? *The American Journal of Occupational Therapy, 71*(3), 7103190050p1–7103190050p9.
52. Gully, S.E. (2018). *Measuring the Effects of Prosthetic Tactile Pacing on Overt Stuttering Frequency in Adults who Stutter* [Thesis]. University of Mississippi, Oxford, Mississippi.
53. Hagg, M. & Larsson, B. (2004). Effects of Motor and Sensory Stimulation in Stroke Patients with Long-Lasting Dysphagia. *Dysphagia, 19,* 219-230.

54. Hagg, M. & Anniko, M. (2008). Lip muscle training in stroke patients with dysphagia. *Acta Oto-Laryngologica, 128,* 1028-1033.
55. Harvard Health Publishing (2016). *Can you grow new brain cells?* Retrieved from https://www.health.harvard.edu/mind-and-mood/can-you-grow-new-brain-cells
56. Harvard Health Publishing. (2019). *9 ways to relieve acid reflux without medication.* Retrieved from https://www.health.harvard.edu/digestive-health/9-ways-to-relieve-acid-reflux-without-medication
57. Healthwise Staff. (2020). *Conserving Energy When You Have COPD or Other Chronic Conditions.* Retrieved from https://myhealth.alberta.ca/Health/Pages/conditions.aspx?hwid=abp2734
58. Heerema, E. (2020). *The Benefits of Routines for People With Dementia: How Consistent Caregivers Can Help in Alzheimer's Disease.* Retrieved from https://www.verywellhealth.com/using-routines-in-dementia-97625
59. Hoag.org. (2012). *Esophageal Soft Diet* [Data file]. Retrieved from https://www.hoag.org/documents/Esophageal-Soft-Diet.pdf
60. Hogan, C.L. (2004). *Stuttering: What It Is, What It Isn't, And What Worked for Me.* Minnesota State University Mankato. Retrieved from https://www.mnsu.edu/comdis/kuster/TherapyWWW/hogan.html
61. Huckabee, M. L., & Steele, C. M. (2006). An analysis of lingual contribution to submental surface electromyographic measures and pharyngeal pressure during effortful swallow. *Archives of Physical Medicine and Rehabilitation, 87,* 1067–1072.
62. The International Dysphagia Standardisation Initiative. (2021). *Resources.* Retrieved from https://iddsi.org/resources/
63. Jewell, T. (2018). *What is Diaphragmatic Breathing?* Healthline Media. Retrieved from https://www.healthline.com/health/diaphragmatic-breathing
64. John Hopkins Medicine. [n.d.-a] *Cleaning and Caring for Tracheostomy Equipment.* Retrieved from https://www.hopkinsmedicine.org/tracheostomy/living/equipment_cleaning.html
65. John Hopkins Medicine. [n.d.-b]. *Tracheostomy and a Passy-Muir Valve.* Retrieved from https://www.hopkinsmedicine.org/tracheostomy/living/passey-muir_valve.html
66. Kalinowski, J., & Saltuklaroglu, T. (2003). Choral speech: the amelioration of stuttering via imitation and the mirror neuronal system. *Neuroscience and Behavioral Reviews, 27*(4) 339-347.
67. Kelly, M.E. & O'Sullivan, M. (2015). *Strategies and Techniques for Cognitive Rehabilitation: Manual for healthcare professionals working with individuals with cognitive impairment* [Data file]. DOI: 10.13140/RG.2.1.1174.3443
68. Kleim, J.A. & Jones, T.A. (2008). Principles of Experience-Dependent Neural Plasticity: Implications for Rehabilitation After Brain Damage. *Journal of Speech, Language, and Hearing Research, 51,* S225-S239.
69. Konecny, P., Elfmark, M., & Urbanek, K. (2011). Facial paresis after stroke and its impact on patients' facial movement and mental status. *Journal of Rehabilitation Medicine, 43,* 73-75.
70. Kotby, M.N., El-Sady, S.R., Basiouny, S.E., Abou-Rass, Y.A., & Hegazi, M.A. (1991). Efficacy of the accent method of voice therapy. *Journal of Voice, 5*(4) 316-320.
71. Kuehn, D.P. (1991). New therapy for treating hypernasal speech using continuous positive airway pressure (CPAP). *Plastic and Reconstructive Surgery, 88,* 959-966.
72. Kuster, J. [n.d.] *Establishment of Light Articulatory Contacts.* Minnesota State University Mankato. Retrieved from http://www.mnsu.edu/comdis/kuster/TherapyWWW/childtherapy/3.html
73. Lombard, L. E., & Steinhauer, K. M. (2007). A novel treatment for hypophonic voice: Twang therapy. *Journal of Voice, 21,* 294–299.
74. Landauer, T.K., & Bjork, R.A. (1978). *Optimum rehearsal patterns and name learning.* In M. Gruneberg, P. E. Morris, & R. N. Sykes (Eds.), Practical aspects of memory (pp. 625–632). London: Academic Press.
75. Langmore, S. E., Terpenning, M. S., Schork, A., Chen, Y., Murray, J. T., Lopatin, D., & Loesche, W. J. (1998). Predictors of aspiration pneumonia: how important is dysphagia? *Dysphagia, 13*(2), 69–81. https://doi.org/10.1007/PL00009559
76. Leonard, C., Rochon, E., & Laird, L. (2008). Treating naming impairment in aphasia: findings from a phonological components analysis treatment. *Aphasiology, 22*(9): 923-947.
77. Logan, K. [n.d.]. *Helping Clients Who Clutter Regular Speaking Rate.* Minnesota State University Mankato. Retrieved https://www.mnsu.edu/comdis/ica1/papers/loganc.html
78. LSVT Global, Inc. (2021). *LSVT LOUD.* Retrieved from https://lsvtglobal.com/lsvtloud
79. Maas, E., Robin, D.A., Hula, S.N.A., Wulf, G., Ballard, K.J., & Schmidt, R.A. (2008). Principles of Motor Learning in Treatment of Motor Speech Disorders. *American Journal of Speech-Language Pathology, 17,* 277-298.
80. Mann, G. (2002). *MASA: The Mann Assessment of Swallowing Ability* [Assessment Instrument]. Clifton Park, NY: Singular.
81. Mawer, R. (2020). *The 18 Best Healthy Foods to Gain Weight Fast.* Healthline Media. Retrieved from https://www.healthline.com/nutrition/18-foods-to-gain-weight

82. Mayo Clinic Staff. (2018). *Hypoxemia*. Retrieved from https://www.mayoclinic.org/symptoms/hypoxemia/basics/definition/sym-20050930
83. Mayo Clinic Staff. (2020). *Gastroesophageal reflux disease (GERD)*. Retrieved from https://www.mayoclinic.org/diseases-conditions/gerd/diagnosis-treatment/drc-20361959
84. Mayo Clinic Staff. (2021). *Memory loss: 7 tips to improve your memory*. Retrieved from https://www.mayoclinic.org/healthy-lifestyle/healthy-aging/in-depth/memory-loss/art-20046518
85. Mckee, A., & Starmer, H. [n.d.] *A practical approach to tracheostomy tubes and ventilators* [Data file]. Retrieved from https://coe.uoregon.edu/cds/files/2019/12/trach-vent-powerpoint.pdf
86. McKenna, V.S., Zhang, B., Haines, M.B., & Kelchner, L.N. (2017). A Systematic Review of Isometric Lingual Strength-Training Programs in Adults With and Without Dysphagia. *American Journal of Speech-Language Pathology, 26*(2), 524-539.
87. MedlinePlus. (2019). *Using an incentive spirometer*. Retrieved from https://medlineplus.gov/ency/patientinstructions/000451.htm
88. Mehta, R., & Zhu R. J. (2009). Blue or Red? Exploring the Effect of Color on Cognitive Task Performances. *Science, 323*(5918), 1226-1229.
89. Maryland Department of Health and Mental Hygiene. (2014). *Maryland Department of Health and Mental Hygiene: Diet Manual for Long-Term Care Residents* [Data File]. Retrieved from https://health.maryland.gov/ohcq/docs/diet_manual_4-3-14.pdf
90. Meerschman, I., D'haeseleer, E., Catry, T. Ruigrok, B., Claeys, S., & Van Lierde, K. (2017). Effect of two isolated vocal facilitating techniques glottal fry and yawn-sigh on the phonation of female speech-language pathology students: A pilot study. *Journal of Communication Disorders, 66*, 40-50.
91. Memorial Sloan Kettering Cancer Center. (2018). *Radiation Therapy to the Head and Neck*. Retrieved from https://www.mskcc.org/cancer-care/patient-education/radiation-therapy-head-and-neck
92. Mills, R.H. (2008). Dysphagia Management: Using Thickened Liquids. *The ASHA Leader, 13*(14), 12-13.
93. Miloro, K.V., Pearson, W.G., Langmore, S.E. (2014). Effortful Pitch Glide: A Potential New Exercise Evaluated by Dynamic MRI. *Journal of Speech, Language, and Hearing Research, 57*(4), 1243-1250.
94. Miranda, V.D.M., Scarpel, R.D., Torres, A.C.M., & Agra, I.M.G. (2015). Effectiveness of speech therapy in patients with facial paralysis after parotidectomy. *Revista CEFAC 17*(3), 984. DOI: https://doi.org/10.1590/1982-021620157314
95. Molt, L., & Yaruss, J.S. (2021). *Neurogenic Stuttering*. The Stuttering Foundation. Retrieved from https://www.stutteringhelp.org/neurogenic-stuttering
96. Namiki, C., Hara, K., Tohara, H., Kobayashi, K., Chantaramanee, A., Nakagawa, K., Saitou, T., Yamaguchi, K., Nakane A., & Minakuchi, S. (2019). Tongue-pressure resistance training improves tongue and supra hyoid muscle functions simultaneously. *Clinical Interventions in Aging, 14*, 601-608. DOI: 10.2147/CIA.S194808
97. The National Aphasia Association. [n.d.-a] *Communication Strategies: Some Do's and Don'ts*. Retrieved from https://www.aphasia.org/aphasia-resources/communication-tips/
98. The National Aphasia Association. [n.d.-b] *That's a Fact! Quick Tips for Aphasia-Friendly Communication (Part Two)*. Retrieved from https://www.aphasia.org/stories/thats-a-fact-quick-tips-for-aphasia-friendly-communication-part-two/
99. National Cancer Institute. (2019). *Oral Complication of Chemotherapy and Head/Neck/Radiation (PDQ®)-Patient Version*. Retrieved from https://www.cancer.gov/about-cancer/treatment/side-effects/mouth-throat/oral-complications-pdq
100. National Institute on Aging. (2017a). *Fall-Proofing Your Home*. Retrieved from https://www.nia.nih.gov/health/fall-proofing-your-home
101. National Institute on Aging. (2017b). *Prevent Falls and Fractures*. Retrieved from https://www.nia.nih.gov/health/prevent-falls-and-fractures
102. National Institute on Aging. (2020). *Cognitive Health and Older Adults*. Retrieved from https://www.nia.nih.gov/health/cognitive-health-and-older-adults
103. National Institute on Deafness and Other Communication Disorders. (2017). *Taking Care of Your Voice*. National Institute on Deafness and Other Communication Disorders. Retrieved from https://www.nidcd.nih.gov/health/taking-care-your-voice
104. Netsell, R.W. (1998). Speech Rehabilitation for Individuals with Unintelligible Speech and Dysarthria: The Respiratory and Velopharyngeal Systems. *Journal of Medical Speech-Language Pathology 6*(2), 107-110.
105. Niemeier, J. (1998). The lighthouse strategy: Use of a visual imagery technique to treat visual inattention in stroke patients. *Brain Injury, 12*(5), 399-406.

106. NSW Government. (2020). *Nasal airflow disorders*. NSW Government. http://www.nchn.org.au/cleft/treatment/nasal_airflow_disords.htm
107. Oza, R., Rundell, K., & Garcellano, M. (2017). Recurrent Ischemic Stroke: Strategies for Prevention. *American Family Physician, 96*(7), 436-440.
108. Panther, K.M. (2005). The Frazier Free Water Protocol. *Perspectives on Swallowing and Swallowing Disorders (Dysphagia) American Speech-Language-Hearing Association Division 13, 4*(1): 4-9.
109. Park, J.S., Oh, D.H., Chang, M.Y., & Kim, K.M. (2016). Effects of expiratory muscle strength training on oropharyngeal dysphagia in subacute stroke patients: a randomised controlled trial. *Journal of Oral Rehabilitation, 43*(5), 364-372.
110. PassyMuir, Inc. [n.d.] *PassyMuir Valves*. Retrieved from www.passy-muir.com
111. Pleton, J. (2015). *Procedure: Passy Muir Valve Placement* [Data file]. Retrieved from https://www.passy-muir.com/wp-content/uploads/2018/10/placement_pmv_madonna.pdf
112. Perlman, A.L., Luschel, E.S., & Du Mond, C.E. (1989). Electrical activity from the superior pharyngeal constrictor during reflexive and nonreflexive tasks. *Journal of Speech, Language, and Hearing Research, 32*(4), 749-754.
113. Pexels. (2021). *Home page*. Retrieved from https://www.pexels.com
114. Pitts, T., Bolser, D., Rosenbeck, J., Troche, M., Okun, M.S., & Sapienza, C. (2009). Impact of Expiratory Muscle Strength Training on Voluntary Cough and Swallow Function in Parkinson Disease. *Chest, 5*, 1301-1308.
115. Pixabay GmbH. (2021). *Home page*. Retrieved from https://pixabay.com
116. Provencio-Arambula, M., Provencio, D., & Hegde, M. N. (2007). Treatment for Oral Phase Dysphagia: Improving Tongue Base Control. In *Treatment of Dysphagia in Adults* (pp. 113-143). San Diego: Plural Publishing, Incorporated.
117. Pruski, A. (2021). *Stroke Recovery Timeline*. The John Hopkins University. Retrieved from https://www.hopkinsmedicine.org/health/conditions-and-diseases/stroke/stroke-recovery-timeline
118. Richard, T. (Host). (2017, November 7). 013 - Rebecca Levy M.S. CCC-SLP - Exercises, Exercises & More Exercises! Evidence-Based Treatment for Every Swallowing Impairment (No. 13). In *Swallow Your Pride*. Mobile Dysphagia Diagnostics Speech-Language Pathology Swallowing Services, P.C. https://www.mobiledysphagiadiagnostics.com/013-rebecca-levy-m-s-ccc-slp-exercises-exercises-more-exercises-evidence-based-treatment-for-every-swallowing-impairment/
119. Robbins, J., Kays, S.A., Gangnon, R.E., Hind, J.A., Hewitt, A.L., Gentry, L.R., & Taylor, A.J. (2007). The Effects of Lingual Exercise in Stroke Patients With Dysphagia. *Archives of Physical Medicine and Rehabilitation, 88*(2), 150-158.
120. Robbins, J., Butler, S.G., Daniels, S.K., Gross, R.D., Langmore, S., Lazarus, C.L., Martin-Harris, B., McCabe, D., Musson, N., & Rosenbek, J.C. (2008). Swallowing and Dysphagia Rehabilitation: Translating Principles of Neural Plasticity Into Clinically Oriented Evidence. *Journal of Speech, Language, and Hearing Research, 51*, S276-300.
121. Rogalski, Y., Edmonds, L., Daly, V., & Gardner, M. (2013). Attentive Reading and Constrained Summarisation (ARCS) discourse treatment for chronic Wernicke's aphasia. *Aphasiology, 27*(10), 1232 – 1251.
122. Rosenbek, J. C., & LaPointe, L. L. (1985). *The dysarthrias: Description, diagnosis, and treatment*. In D. Johns (Ed.), Clinical management of neurogenic communication disorders (pp. 97-152). Boston: Little Brown.
123. Roy, N., & Leeper, H.A. (1993). Effects of the manual laryngeal musculoskeletal tension reduction technique as a treatment for functional voice disorders: perceptual and acoustic measures. *Journal of Voice, 7*(3), 242–249.
124. Saconato, M., Chiari, B.M., Lederman, H.M., & Goncalves, M.I.R. (2016). Effectiveness of Chin-tuck Maneuver to Facilitate Swallowing in Neurologic Dysphagia. *International Archives of Otorhinolaryngology, 20*(1), 13-17.
125. Santini, C. (n.d.) *Facial Paralysis due to Peripheral Nerve Injury - SLP evaluation and treatment* [Data File]. Retrieved from https://cdn.ymaws.com/www.flasha.org/resource/resmgr/session2018.pdf
126. Sapienza, C.M., & Wheeler, K. (2006). Respiratory muscle strength training: functional outcomes versus plasticity. *Seminars in Speech and Language, 27*(4), 236-244.
127. Shaker, R., Kern, M, Bardan, E. Taylor, A., Stewart, E.T., Arndorder, R.C., Hoffman, R.G., & Bonnevier, J. (1997). Augmentation of deglutitive upper esophageal sphincter opening in the elderly by exercise. *American Journal of Physiology, 272*(6), G1518-G1522.
128. Smania, N., Bazoli, F., Piva, D., & Guidetti, G. (1997). Visuomotor Imagery and Rehabilitation of Neglect. *Archives of Physical Medicine and Rehabilitation, 78*, 430-436.
129. Sohlberg, M.M., Ehlhardt, L., & Kennedy, M. (2005). Instructional Techniques in Cognitive Rehabilitation: A Preliminary Report. *Seminars in Speech and Language, 26*(4), 268-279.
130. Stemple, J.C. (n.d.) *Chapter Three: Learning/Teaching Vocal Function Exercise* [Online lecture]. MedBridge, Inc. https://www.medbridgeeducation.com/courses/details/vocal-function-exercises-joseph-stemple-speech-langauge-pathology-vocal-therapy

131. Stevens, J.H. (2011) *Eating and Swallowing Guidelines* [Data file]. Washington State Department of Social and Health Services. Retrieved from https://www.dshs.wa.gov/sites/default/files/DDA/dda/documents/Eating%20Swallowing%20Guidelines.pdf
132. Stroke Association. (n.d.) *Headaches after stroke*. Retrieved from https://www.stroke.org.uk/effects-of-stroke/physical-effects-of-stroke/pain-and-headaches
133. Sulica, L. (2010). Clinical characteristics of essential voice tremor: a study of 34 cases. *Laryngoscope, 120*(3), 516-528.
134. Sura, L., Madhavan, A., Carnaby, G.D., & Crary, M.A. (2012). Dysphagia in the elderly: management and nutritional considerations. *Clinical Interventions in Aging, 7*, 287-298.
135. Sutton, M. (2014). *What is Left Neglect?* Tactus Therapy. Retrieved from https://tactustherapy.com/what-is-left-neglect/
136. Swanberg, M.M, Nasreddine, Z.S., Mendez, M.F., & Cummings, J.L. (2007). Chapter 6: Speech and Language (pp.79-98). In C.G. Goetz (Ed.), *Clinical Neurology (third edition)*. Saunders Elsevier.
137. Tabor, L., Plowman, E., & Martin, K. (2017). *Living With ALS Resource Guide 8: Adjusting to Swallowing Changes and Nutritional Management in ALS* [Data File]. Retrieved from https://www.neals.org/uploads/blog/doc/Swallowing_Changes_in_ALS.pdf
138. Tan, C., Liu, Y., Li.W., Liu, J., & Chen, L. (2013). Transcutaneous neuromuscular electrical stimulation can improve swallowing function in patients with dysphagia caused by non-stroke diseases: a meta-analysis. *Journal of Oral Rehabilitation, 40*(6), 472-480.
139. Thompson, C.K. & Shapiro, L.P. (2005.) Treating agrammatic aphasia within a linguistic framework: Treatment of Underlying Forms. *Aphasiology, 19*, 1021–1036.
140. Van Nuffelen, G., De Bodt, M., Wuyts, F., & Van de Heyning, P. (2009). The Effect of Rate Control on Speech Rate and Intelligibility of Dysarthric Speech. *Folia Phoniatrica et Logopaedica, 61*, 69-75.
141. Vaughan, A., Gardner, D., Miles, A., Copley, A., Wenke, R., & Coulson, S. (2020). A Systematic Review of Physical Rehabilitation of Facial Palsy. *Frontiers in Neurology, 11*, 222.
142. The Voice Foundation. [n.d.] *Myasthenia Gravis (MG)*. The Voice Foundation. Retrieved from https://voicefoundation.org/health-science/voice-disorders/voice-disorders/voice-dysfunction-in-neurological-disorders/myasthenia-gravis-mg/#:~:text=Some%20laryngologists%20have%20described%20%E2%80%9Cisolated,jaw%2C%20or%20facial%20muscular%20weakness.
143. Wambaugh, J. (2003). A comparison of the relative effects of phonologic and semantic cueing treatments. *Aphasiology, 17*(5), 433-441.
144. Wambaugh, J.L., & Mausycki, S.C. (2010). Sound Production Treatment: Application with severe apraxia of speech. *Aphasiology, 24*(6-8), 814-825. DOI: 10.1080/02687030903422494
145. Watts, C.R., Hamilton, A., Toles, L., Childs, L., & Mau, T. (2015). A randomized controlled trial of stretch-and-flow voice therapy for muscle tension Dysphonia. *The Laryngoscope, 125*(6), 1420-1425. https://doi.org/10.1002/lary.25155
146. Yoon, W.L., Khoo, J.K., & Rickard Liow, S.J. (2014). Chin tuck against resistance (CTAR): new method for enhancing suprahyoid muscle activity using a Shaker-type exercise. *Dysphagia, 29*(2), 243-248.

About the Author

Chung Hwa is an author, artist, speech-language pathologist, and visiting professor at Western Washington University's Department of Communication Sciences and Disorders.

Chung Hwa has worked with adults in all stages of recovery, from the ICU, to SNFs, home health, outpatient, and telehealth. She and her sister (an occupational therapist and the editor of this book!) created **theadultspeechtherapyworkbook.com** where you can find a printable version of this workbook, Assessment Templates, Goal Banks, Documentation Guides, plus many free resources.

Chung Hwa lives in Washington state with her family.

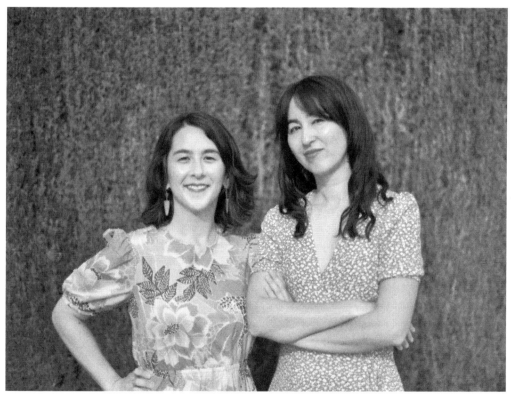

The author and the editor.